Late Life Depression

Editor

W. VAUGHN MCCALL

PSYCHIATRIC CLINICS OF NORTH AMERICA

www.psych.theclinics.com

December 2013 • Volume 36 • Number 4

ELSEVIER

1600 John F. Kennedy Boulevard • Suite 1800 • Philadelphia, Pennsylvania, 19103-2899

http://www.theclinics.com

PSYCHIATRIC CLINICS OF NORTH AMERICA Volume 36, Number 4
December 2013 ISSN 0193-953X, ISBN-13: 978-0-323-26124-1

Editor: Joanne Husovski
Developmental Editor: Stephanie Carter

Psychiatric Clinics of North America (ISSN 0193-953X) is published quarterly by Elsevier Inc., 360 Park Avenue South, New York, NY 10010-1710. Months of issue are March, June, September, and December. Business and Editorial Offices: 1600 John F. Kennedy Blvd., Suite 1800, Philadelphia, PA 19103-2899. Periodicals postage paid at New York, NY and additional mailing offices. Subscription prices are $300.00 per year (US individuals), $546.00 per year (US institutions), $150.00 per year (US students/residents), $365.00 per year (Canadian individuals), $687.00 per year (Canadian Institutions), $455.00 per year (foreign individuals), $687.00 per year (foreign institutions), and $220.00 per year (international & Canadian students/residents). Foreign air speed delivery is included in all *Clinics'* subscription prices. All prices are subject to change without notice. **POSTMASTER:** Send address changes to *Psychiatric Clinics of North America*, Elsevier Health Sciences Division, Subscription Customer Service, 3251 Riverport Lane, Maryland Heights, MO 63043. Customer Service: 1-800-654-2452 (US). From outside the United States, call 1-314-447-8871. Fax: 1-314-447-8029. E-mail: journalscustomerservice-usa@elsevier.com (for print support) and journalsonlinesupport-usa@elsevier.com (for online support).

Reprints. For copies of 100 or more, of articles in this publication, please contact the Commercial Reprints Department, Elsevier Inc., 360 Park Avenue South, New York, New York 10010-1710. Tel.: 212-633-3874, Fax: 212-633-3820, E-mail: reprints@elsevier.com.

Psychiatric Clinics of North America is covered in *MEDLINE/PubMed (Index Medicus), Current Contents/Social and Behavioral Sciences, Social Science Citation Index, Embase/Excerpta Medica,* and PsycINFO.

Printed and bound by CPI Group (UK) Ltd, Croydon, CR0 4YY

Transferred to digital print 2012

Contributors

EDITOR

W. VAUGHN MCCALL, MD, MS
Case Distinguished Chair and Professor, Department of Psychiatry and Health Behavior, Medical College of Georgia, Georgia Regents University of Augusta, Augusta, Georgia

AUTHORS

GEORGE S. ALEXOPOULOS, MD
Stephen P. Tobin and Dr Arnold M. Cooper Professor of Psychiatry, Institute of Geriatric Psychiatry, Weill Cornell Medical College, White Plains, New York

REHAN AZIZ, MD
Department of Psychiatry, Institute of Living, Hartford Hospital, Hartford; Assistant Clinical Professor of Psychiatry, Department of Psychiatry, Yale University School of Medicine, New Haven; Assistant Professor of Psychiatry, Department of Psychiatry, University of Connecticut Health Center, Farmington, Connecticut

JEANNE M. CARTIER, PhD, PMHCNS-BC, CNE
Associate Professor, Interim Program Director, DNP-Primary Care, Department of Biobehavioral Nursing, College of Nursing, Georgia Regents University, Augusta, Georgia

JAMES DOORLEY, BA
Depression Clinical and Research Program, Department of Psychiatry, Massachusetts General Hospital, Harvard Medical School, Boston, Massachusetts

KELLEY DURHAM, BA
Depression Clinical and Research Program, Department of Psychiatry, Massachusetts General Hospital, Harvard Medical School, Boston, Massachusetts

CORINNE FISCHER, MD
Department of Psychiatry, Li Ka Shing Knowledge Institute, St. Michael's Hospital, University of Toronto, Toronto, Ontario, Canada

JENNIFER L. FRANCIS, PhD
Assistant Professor of Clinical Psychiatry, Department of Psychiatry, University of Illinois at Chicago, Chicago, Illinois

MARLENE P. FREEMAN, MD
Perinatal and Reproductive Psychiatry Program, Department of Psychiatry, Massachusetts General Hospital, Harvard Medical School, Boston, Massachusetts

ONDRIA C. GLEASON, MD
Interim Dean, School of Community Medicine; Professor and Chair, Department of Psychiatry, The University of Oklahoma School of Community Medicine, Tulsa, Oklahoma

JULIET GLOVER, MD
Geriatric Psychiatry Fellow, Palmetto Health, University of South Carolina School of
Medicine, Columbia, South Carolina

ADRIANA P. HERMIDA, MD
Assistant Professor, Department of Psychiatry and Behavioral Sciences, Emory
University, Atlanta, Georgia

ZAHINOOR ISMAIL, MD, FRCPC
Clinical Associate Professor of Psychiatry and Neurology, Hotchkiss Brain Institute,
University of Calgary, Calgary, Alberta; Assistant Professor University of Toronto,
Toronto, Ontario, Canada

KRISTINA W. KINTZIGER, PhD
Assistant Professor, Department of Biostatistics and Epidemiology, Medical College of
Georgia, Georgia Regents University, Augusta, Georgia

ROB M. KOK, MD, PhD
Department of Old Age Psychiatry, Parnassia Psychiatric Institute, The Hague,
The Netherlands

ANAND KUMAR, MD
Lizzie Gilman Professor and Head, Department of Psychiatry, University of Illinois at
Chicago, Chicago, Illinois

W. VAUGHN MCCALL, MD, MS
Case Distinguished Chair and Professor, Department of Psychiatry and Health Behavior,
Medical College of Georgia, Georgia Regents University of Augusta, Augusta, Georgia

WILLIAM M. MCDONALD, MD
Professor, JB Fuqua Chair for Late-Life Depression, Director, Department of Psychiatry
and Behavioral Sciences, Fuqua Center for Late-Life Depression, Emory University,
Atlanta, Georgia

DAVID MISCHOULON, MD, PhD
Depression Clinical and Research Program, Department of Psychiatry, Massachusetts
General Hospital, Harvard Medical School, Boston, Massachusetts

SARAH SHIZUKO MORIMOTO, PsyD
Assistant Professor of Psychology in Psychiatry, Institute of Geriatric Psychiatry, Weill
Cornell Medical College, White Plains, New York

MAREN NYER, PhD
Depression Clinical and Research Program, Department of Psychiatry, Massachusetts
General Hospital, Harvard Medical School, Boston, Massachusetts

AARON M. PIERCE, DO
Assistant Professor, Department of Psychiatry, The University of Oklahoma School of
Community Medicine, Tulsa, Oklahoma

PATRICIO RIVA-POSSE, MD
Assistant Professor, Department of Psychiatry and Behavioral Sciences, Emory
University, Atlanta, Georgia

OLA ROSTANT, PhD
Department of Psychiatry, University of Michigan Medical School, Ann Arbor, Michigan

SHILPA SRINIVASAN, MD, DFAPA
Associate Professor of Clinical Psychiatry, Department of Neuropsychiatry and Behavioral Sciences, University of South Carolina School of Medicine, Columbia, South Carolina

DAVID C. STEFFENS, MD, MHS
Professor and Chairman, Department of Psychiatry, University of Connecticut Health Center, Farmington, Connecticut

ASHLEY E. WALKER, MD
Assistant Professor, Department of Psychiatry, The University of Oklahoma School of Community Medicine, Tulsa, Oklahoma

JULIA K. WARNOCK, MD
Professor, Department of Psychiatry, The University of Oklahoma School of Community Medicine, Tulsa, Oklahoma

TRACY WHARTON, PhD
Department of Psychiatry, University of Michigan Medical School, Ann Arbor, Michigan

ALBERT S. YEUNG, MD, ScD
Depression Clinical and Research Program, Department of Psychiatry, Massachusetts General Hospital, Harvard Medical School, Boston, Massachusetts

KARA ZIVIN, PhD
Serious Mental Illness Treatment Resource and Evaluation Center, Center for Clinical Management Research, Department of Veterans Affairs; Department of Psychiatry, Institute for Social Research, University of Michigan Medical School, Ann Arbor, Michigan

Contents

> Mental health disorders in terms of an aging population are discussed in this review. Statistics on depression in later life are presented with a discussion of physical health comorbidities. This presentation postulates that the health care infrastructure currently in place is inadequate to meet the present, much less the future, needs of this population. The care of the depressed elder will require the coordinated effort of psychiatrists, psychologists, social workers, nurse practitioners and advanced practice psychiatric nurses, internal medicine gerontologists, internal medicine and family medicine general physicians, community agencies, and volunteers.

> This article analyzes late-life depression, looking carefully at what defines a person as *elderly*, the incidence of late-life depression, complications and differences in symptoms between young and old patients with depression, subsyndromal depression, bipolar depression in the elderly, the relationship between grief and depression, along with sleep disturbances and suicidal ideation.

> Although depression in old age is less common than depression in younger populations, it still affects more than 1 million community-living older adults. Depression in late life has been associated with reduced quality of life and increased mortality from both suicide and illness. Its causes are multifactorial but are prominently related to both biologic and social factors. Psychological factors, although less studied in elders, are also important in understanding its cause. In this article, multiple facets of late-life depression are reviewed, including its clinical presentation, epidemiology, and biopsychosocial causes.

> The purpose of this article is to identify the cognitive deficits commonly associated with geriatric depression and describe their clinical significance.

PSYCHIATRIC CLINICS OF NORTH AMERICA

FORTHCOMING ISSUES

March 2014
Neuropsychiatry of Traumatic Brain Injury
Ricardo Jorge, MD, and
David B. Arciniegas, MD, *Editors*

June 2014
Obsessive Compulsive Disorder
Wayne Goodman, MD, *Editor*

September 2014
Sexual Deviance: Assessment and Treatment
John Bradford, MD, and
A.G. Ahmad, MD, *Editors*

RECENT ISSUES

September 2013
Disaster Mental Health: Around the World and Across Time
Craig L. Katz, MD, and
Anand Pandya, MD, *Editors*

June 2013
Psychiatric Manifestations of Neurotoxins
Daniel E. Rusyniak, MD, and
Michael R. Dobbs, MD, *Editors*

March 2013
Complementary and Integrative Therapies for Psychiatric Disorders
Philip R. Muskin, MD,
Patricia L. Gerbarg, MD, and
Richard P. Brown, MD, *Editors*

RELATED INTEREST

Psychiatric Clinics of North America
June 2011 (Vol. 34, No. 4)
Geriatric Psychiatry: Advances and Directions
George S. Alexopoulos, MD, and Dimitri N. Kiosses, PhD, *Editors*

Preface

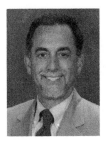

W. Vaughn McCall, MD, MS
Editor

This issue of *Psychiatric Clinics of North America* is devoted to Late Life Depression. As revealed in this issue, there is much to be hopeful about. We have an improved understanding regarding the risks for late life depression, the symptomatic presentation, the complications, the etiology, and the treatment response. On the other hand, there is also much to be concerned about. The vast improvement in understanding late life depression will be of only theoretical value if there are an insufficient number of caregivers to deliver the care that is necessary. We are witnessing a dangerous confluence of two factors—a burgeoning growth of elders around the world, while the number of trained geriatric providers shrinks in absolute numbers. For these reasons, the content of this issue is directed not only to geriatric specialists of all stripes but also to primary care providers and non-geriatric-focused specialists, as they will have to carry an increasing share of the work that will need to be done.

W. Vaughn McCall, MD, MS
Case Distinguished Chair and Professor
Department of Psychiatry and Health Behavior
Medical College of Georgia
Georgia Regents University of Augusta, 997 St. Sebastian Way
Augusta, GA 30909, USA

E-mail address:
wmccall@gru.edu

Psychiatr Clin N Am 36 (2013) xi
http://dx.doi.org/10.1016/j.psc.2013.08.011
0193-953X/13/$ – see front matter © 2013 Published by Elsevier Inc.

psych.theclinics.com

Erratum

In the September 2013 issue of *Psychiatric Clinics of North America*, an error is present on page 444 in the article by Raviola et al, "The 2010 Haiti Earthquake Response". The following statement – *A working group composed of representatives from MSPP, the xxx psychiatric hospitals, local and international NGOs, and WHO/PAHO was convened through the cluster in the second half of 2010 with the goal of establishing initial steps toward a national policy and plan for mental health.* "xxx" was unintentionally inserted.

Psychiatr Clin N Am 36 (2013) xiii
http://dx.doi.org/10.1016/j.psc.2013.08.013
psych.theclinics.com

Late Life Depression
A Global Problem with Few Resources

W. Vaughn McCall, MD, MS[a],*, Kristina W. Kintziger, PhD[b]

KEYWORDS

- Late life depression • Aging population • Depressive symptoms
- Health care resources

KEY POINTS

- Depressive disorders are debilitating health problems that are the leading cause of disability worldwide.
- Depressive disorders are associated with greater morbidity and mortality, in general, in older individuals.
- Aging has led to an increase in prevalence and mortality due to noncommunicable chronic conditions worldwide.

AN AGING POPULATION

According to recent United States Census Bureau estimates, more than 41 million (13.3%) individuals were 65 years of age or older in 2011 (**Fig. 1**). Trends suggest that the population in this age group will have increased to more than 92 million, or 21.9% of the population, by 2060 (**Fig. 2**),[1] with 1 in 5 individuals being aged 65 years or older by 2030.[2] In addition, the age structure among those 65 years and older will also shift as the baby boomer generation ages. In 2010, only 14% of those 65 years and older was in the oldest age category (85 years and older). By 2050, the proportion in this age category over 85 years will be 21%.[2]

Similar trends have been noted internationally. The median life expectancy worldwide has increased from 68 years in 1990 to 72 years in 2009 (range: 47–83 years).[3] Data from other developed countries such as Australia, Canada, Japan, and many countries of the European Union also suggest that the average age of these populations is increasing, while fertility rates have declined.[4] Some of these countries are expecting their aging population to increase rapidly over the next 10 years, such as Japan (54%) and Canada (43%), compared to the United States (33%).[4] However,

[a] Department of Psychiatry and Health Behavior, Medical College of Georgia, Georgia Regents University, 997 St. Sebastian Way, Augusta, GA 30909, USA; [b] Department of Biostatistics and Epidemiology, Medical College of Georgia, Georgia Regents University, 1120 15th Street, AE-1005, Augusta, GA 30912, USA
* Corresponding author.
E-mail address: wmccall@gru.edu

Psychiatr Clin N Am 36 (2013) 475–481
http://dx.doi.org/10.1016/j.psc.2013.07.001
0193-953X/13/$ – see front matter © 2013 Elsevier Inc. All rights reserved.

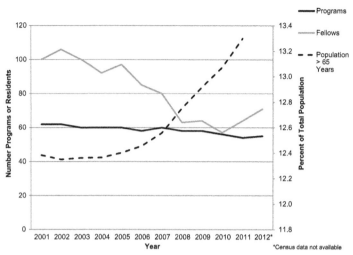

Fig. 1. Number of US geriatric psychiatry programs and fellows with percentage of US population 65 years and older, 2001-2012.

the United States surpasses average global estimates in terms of aging, with 18% of the US population aged 60 and older compared with the average 11%, according to the World Health Organization (WHO).[3]

THE BURDEN OF MENTAL HEALTH DISORDERS
General Mental Health

The WHO estimates that mental health disorders are the most common cause of disabilities in people worldwide. Neuropsychiatric disorders caused about a third of all years lost due to disability (YLDs) in 2004. Furthermore, there is a greater burden of mental health problems in women, with mental disorders making up 3 of the top 10

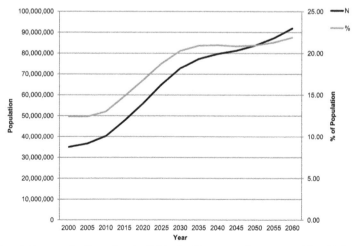

Fig. 2. Population projections for individuals 65 years of age or older, United States, 2000-2060.

leading causes of disease burden for women in low- to mid-income countries, and 4 of the top 10 for women in high-income countries.[5]

The World Mental Health Survey is a survey of mental health problems conducted in 17 countries from 2001 through 2003.[6] Based on the results of this study, the United States has the highest prevalence of mental illness (26.4%) compared with global estimates. Other countries range from 4.3% (Shanghai, China) to 20.5% (Ukraine). Internationally, anxiety (2.4%–18.2%) and mood (0.8%–9.6%) disorders are the most important contributing factors, and most disorders are classified as mild to moderate severity.[6]

In the United States, the Centers for Disease Control and Prevention conducts annual health surveys that collect general information on mental health. The National Health Interview Survey collects information on selected mental health characteristics. In 2011, the overall age-adjusted percentage of individuals who reported experiencing the following symptoms all or some of the time, respectively, is as follows:

- Sadness (3.2/8.6%)
- Hopelessness (2.2/4.5%)
- Worthlessness (1.9/3.5%)
- "Everything is an effort" (5.7/9.2%)

Individuals aged 65 to 74 years and 75 years and older reported similar trends, with those who reported feeling sadness some of the time (9.3% for 65–74 years, and 9.0% for 75 years and older) being higher than the national average.[7]

Depression

Depressive disorders are debilitating health problems that are the leading cause of disability worldwide.[5,8] These disorders are characterized by loss of interest in activities, changes in weight and sleeping patterns, fatigue, and feelings of guilt and worthlessness.[9] Depression can lead to impairments in one's ability to function socially, decreased quality of life, and increased risk of health problems.[10] Finally, it is one of the most common chronic diseases in the general population.[10] In 2000, it was estimated that depression cost the United States $83.1 billion in economic costs, including $26.1 billion in direct health care costs and $51.5 billion in workplace costs based on absenteeism.[11]

Estimates vary regarding rates of depression and depressive symptoms in the United States by source. During 2005 to 2006, the National Health and Nutrition Examination Survey (NHANES) reported that greater than 5% of individuals in the United States experienced depression. These rates varied by age, gender, race/ethnicity, and socioeconomic status.[12] Based on the 2006 and 2008 Behavioral Risk Factor Surveillance System, 9.1% of the US population met the criteria for depression.[13] This survey also showed differences in rates of depression by age, gender, race/ethnicity, and socioeconomic status. In both surveys, depression increased with age, with those between the ages of about 40 and 64 years old having the highest prevalence of depression. Women were more likely to have symptoms of depression than men, and non-Hispanic white individuals were less likely to report depression than individuals of other racial or ethnic groups.[12,13] Low income,[12] low education, unemployed status, and having no health insurance were also related to higher rates of depression.[13] Of individuals reporting symptoms of depression, 80% reported functional impairment. Less than half of these reported contacting a physician or mental health professional for their symptoms.[12]

Among the US population aged 65 years and older, 4.1% reported major depression, 5.1% reported other depression, and 9.1% reported any depression in 2006, according to NHANES.[13] In 2010, it was estimated that between 1.2 and 1.8 million adults 65 years of age and older had a depressive disorder, or 3.0% to 4.5% of this age group. Rates of depressive disorders in community-dwelling elderly persons over the age of 65 vary by race/ethnicity, with the highest rates of depressive disorders being among the Hispanic/Latino populations. Older whites, African-Americans, and Asians report rates of depressive disorders about 3.6% to 4.0%, but older Hispanics report rates of 6.9%. Among individuals in this age group who are in nursing homes, the prevalence of depression is significantly higher (49.6%).[14]

According to NHANES data from 2005 through 2010, 61.72% of individuals aged 65 years and older reported having at least one symptom of depression in the 2-week period before the survey (**Table 1**). The most common symptoms reported in this age group include "feeling tired or having little energy," "trouble sleeping or sleeping too much," "little interest in doing things," and "feeling down, depressed, or hopeless" (**Table 2**). Of those with at least one symptom of depression, 23.72% reported that their symptoms caused them some to extreme difficulty in their daily lives.

Depressive disorders are associated with greater morbidity and mortality, in general, in older individuals. Depression often coexists with other chronic medical conditions in this age population. For example, the highest prevalence for coexisting chronic conditions includes hypertension (58%), chronic pain, and arthritis (56%). Another study showed that individuals over 55 years of age were 4 times more likely to die over a 15-month period than individuals without major depressive disorder.[14]

Globally, it is estimated that 350 million individuals suffer from depression, with 1 in every 20 people having at least one episode of depression in the previous year.[8] Not surprisingly, depression is also the leading cause of disability worldwide, as measured by YLD, in both developed and developing countries.[5,8] Unipolar depressive disorders ranked third worldwide, eighth in low-income countries, and first in both mid- and high-income countries in terms of YLDs. Furthermore, depression was the most common cause among the neuropsychiatric disorders for both men and women, with women having a 50% greater burden of depression than men.[5]

Table 1
Frequency of reported symptoms of depression in adults 65 years of age and older, NHANES depression screener, United States, 2005–2010

Number of Symptoms Reported	%
0	38.28
1	22.07
2	16.27
3	8.57
4	6.42
5	4.07
6	2.64
7	1.14
8	0.40
9	0.14

Responses were weighted to account for sampling design and combining multiple survey years, according to NHANES analytic guidelines.

Data from Centers for Disease Control and Prevention (CDC), National Center for Health Statistics (NCHS). National health and nutrition examination survey data. Hyattsville (MD): US Department of Health and Human Services, CDC. 2005–2010. Available at: http://www.cdc.gov/nchs/nhanes/nhanes_questionnaires.htm. Accessed February, 2013.

Table 2
Categories of reported symptoms of depression in adults 65 years of age and older, NHANES depression screener, United States, 2005–2010

	Did Not Experience Symptom (%)	Did Experience Symptom (%)	Several Days (%)	More Than 1/2 the Days (%)	Nearly Every Day (%)
Little interest in doing things	82.02	17.98	13.31	2.47	2.19
Feeling down, depressed, or hopeless	82.98	17.02	12.67	2.32	2.03
Trouble sleeping or sleeping too much	65.61	34.39	20.18	5.60	8.62
Feeling tired or having little energy	56.88	43.12	27.30	7.13	8.69
Poor appetite or overeating	85.86	14.14	8.64	2.80	2.69
Feeling bad about yourself	90.73	9.27	7.21	0.89	1.17
Trouble concentrating on things	90.19	9.81	6.73	1.16	1.92
Moving or speaking slowly or too fast	93.60	6.40	4.44	0.99	0.97
Thought you would be better off dead	97.55	2.45	1.87	0.28	0.31

Responses were weighted to account for sampling design and combining multiple survey years, according to NHANES analytic guidelines.

Data from Centers for Disease Control and Prevention (CDC), National Center for Health Statistics (NCHS). National health and nutrition examination survey data. Hyattsville (MD): US Department of Health and Human Services, CDC. 2005–2010. Available at: http://www.cdc.gov/nchs/nhanes/nhanes_questionnaires.htm. Accessed February, 2013.

IMPACT OF AGING ON HEALTH CARE RESOURCES
General Health Care Resources

With the growing population aged 65 years and over and the longer life expectancy of individuals, the demand on health care services by the geriatric populations is expected to increase. Understanding how this demand will affect both general and specialized medical care is important for planning in terms of manpower and resources.

Aging has led to an increase in prevalence and mortality due to noncommunicable chronic conditions worldwide.[3] Furthermore, as individuals age, their health care utilization increases, starting around age 55.[15] One study suggests that population aging will have a modest effect on total hospital utilization. From 2005 to 2015, aging will account for a 7.6% increase on per person inpatient resources, or 0.74% per year. This amount is more than double the increase in demand from the previous 10-year period (0.35% per year increase).[15]

Although there are a large number of family and general internal medicine physicians in the United States (about 208,000 in 2008), there are few physicians with specialized training to deal with the demands of this ever-increasing population. Of the medical programs surveyed in 2008, about half of family medicine and one-third of internal medicine residency programs offered 12 or fewer hours of specific geriatric training to their residents. In 2011, there were only about 7500 board-certified geriatricians in the United States. Although there may be adequate residency programs available for geriatric medicine, between one-fourth and one-half of fellowship positions have not been filled annually over the past 20 years.[14]

Mental Health Resources

In general, there are limited resources worldwide and nationally to deal with mental illness in terms of both manpower and infrastructure. According to WHO estimates, there are only 0.3 (global) and 0.8 (US) psychiatrists per 10,000 population, and 2.5 (global) and 3.4 (US) psychiatric hospital beds per 10,000 population. In the European region, there are 1.1 psychiatrists and 6.3 psychiatric beds per 10,000 population.[3] These statistics demonstrate that the United States is lagging in terms of focused mental health care professionals and resources.

The situation is far worse for specialized psychiatric care of the aging population. In 2012, there were 1707 active board-certified geriatric psychiatrists, 55 accredited geriatric psychiatry programs, and 71 geriatric psychiatry fellows in the United States (American Board of Psychiatry and Neurology, personal communication, 2013). Therefore, there are approximately 0.4 geriatric psychiatrists per 10,000 population aged 65 and over (**Fig. 3**). A recent Institute of Medicine report focused on mental health care of the aging population in the United States. The number of geriatric psychiatrists has remained fairly stable over the past 20 years.[14] If the population increases as expected, and the number of specialists remains relatively stable over this time, there will be 0.2 geriatric psychiatrists per 10,000 population aged 65 and older in 2060. Furthermore, based on the way that health care services have evolved, it is difficult to predict with accuracy the number of specialists that will be needed in the future to care for this population.[14] In addition to the specialized mental health or geriatric physicians, there are about 9000 registered nurses specialized in gerontology, 19,000 registered nurses specialized in mental health, and 1700 geriatric pharmacists. Finally, starting in 2011, physician assistants are able to be certified in certain areas of psychiatry.[14]

As the population ages, it is obvious that there will be a greater demand on health care resources by those 65 years of age and older. The infrastructure that is currently in place is inadequate to meet the present, much less the future, needs of this population. A greater emphasis must be placed on the challenges of aging, and specifically, the mental health problems of aging, in terms of infrastructure, resources, personnel, and training programs to manage and treat late life depression successfully. The care of the depressed elder will necessarily require the coordinated effort of general

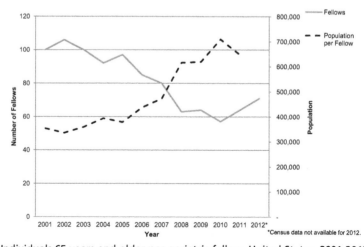

Fig. 3. Individuals 65 years and older per geriatric fellow, United States, 2001-2012.

psychiatrists (a few), geriatric psychiatrists, general and geriatric psychologists, social workers, nurse practitioners and advanced practice psychiatric nurses, internal medicine gerontologists, internal medicine and family medicine general physicians, community agencies, and volunteers.

REFERENCES

1. United States Census Bureau: American FactFinder [US Census Bureau]. 2013. Available at: www.census.gov. Accessed January 2, 2013.
2. Vincent GK, Velkoff VA. The next four decades - the older population in the United States: 2010 to 2050. Washington, DC: US Department of Commerce, Economics and Statististics Administration, US Census Bureau; 2010. Current Population Reports. 1-2-2013.
3. World health statistics 2012. Geneva (Switzerland): World Health Organization; 2012.
4. Anderson GF, Hussey PS. Population aging: a comparison among industrialized countries. Health Aff 2000;19(3):191–203.
5. The global burden of disease 2004 update. Geneva (Switzerland): World Health Organization; 2004.
6. Demyttenaere K, Bruffaerts R, Posada-Villa J, et al. Prevalence, severity, and unmet need for treatment of mental disorders in the World Health Organization World Mental Health Surveys. JAMA 2004;291(21):2581–90.
7. Summary health statistics for US adults: National Health Interview Survey, 2011. Series 10, Number 256. 2012. Hyattsville (MD), National Center for Health Statistics, Centers for Disease Control and Prevention.
8. Marcus M, Yasamy MT, van Ommeren M, et al. Depression: a global public health concern. Geneva (Switzerland): World Health Organization; 2012. 1-2-2013.
9. American Psychiatric Association: Diagnostic and Statistical Manual of Mental Disorders. Fifth Edition. Arlington, VA: American Psychiatric Association; 2013.
10. Wang PS, Simon G, Kessler RC. The economic burden of depression and the cost-effectiveness of treatment. Int J Methods Psychiatr Res 2003;12(1):22–33.
11. Greenberg PE, Kessler RC, Birnbaum HG, et al. The economic burden of depression in the United States: how did it change between 1990 and 2000? J Clin Psychiatry 2003;64(12):1465–75.
12. Pratt LA, Brody DJ. Depression in the United States Household Population, 2005-2006, vol. 7. Atlanta (GA): Centers for Disease Control and Prevention; 2008. NCHS Data Brief. 1-2-2013.
13. Gonzalez O, McKnight-Eily LR, Strine T, et al. Current depression among adults—United States, 2006 and 2008. MMWR Morb Mortal Wkly Rep 2010;59(38): 1229–35.
14. IOM (Institute of Medicine). The mental health and substance abuse workforce for older adults: In whose hands? Washington, DC: The National Academies Press; 2012.
15. Strunk BC, Ginsburg PB, Banker MI. The effect of population aging on future hospital demand. Health Aff 2006;25(3):w141–9.

What Characterizes Late-Life Depression?

Zahinoor Ismail, MD, FRCPC[a,b,]*, Corinne Fischer, MD[c],
W. Vaughn McCall, MD, MS[d]

KEYWORDS

- Late-life depression • Complications in depression • Bipolar • Sleep disturbance
- Suicide • Geriatric medicine

KEY POINTS

- Only relatively recently has it become accepted that some of the decline associated with aging is caused by disease processes and that successful aging is possible.
- Confounding prevalence and incidence estimates of late-life depression is the finding that depression has a variable course and trajectory in older adults.
- Late-life depression is associated with higher levels of medical comorbidity, cognitive impairment, and mortality and has a bidirectional relationship with frailty.
- Overlap between apathy and depression is an area of controversy, given that patients with apathy may be wrongly diagnosed with depression.
- In terms of common comorbidities, studies have recently shown that late-life bipolar affective disorder is commonly comorbid with alcohol abuse, panic attacks, generalized anxiety disorder, and dysthymia.

WHO ARE THE ELDERLY?

Aging is a dynamic concept that has changed throughout history as a result of demographic changes and the acquisition of new knowledge. Before the mid-1970s, it was thought that aging was associated primarily with an inexorable decline in physical and cognitive functions. Only relatively recently has it become accepted that some of the decline associated with aging is caused by disease processes and that successful aging is possible.[1] This acceptance ushered in policy changes that led to the development of geriatric-specific services.[2] Life expectancy has also affected our impression

[a] Hotchkiss Brain Institute, University of Calgary, 1402 29 St NW, Calgary, Alberta, Canada T2N 2T9; [b] University of Toronto, Toronto, Ontario, Canada; [c] Li Ka Shing Knowledge Institute, St Michael's Hospital, Department of Psychiatry, University of Toronto, Room 17044cc Wing, #30 Bond Street, Toronto, Ontario, Canada M5B 1W8; [d] Department of Psychiatry and Health Behavior, Medical College of Georgia, Georgia Regents University of Augusta, Augusta, GA, USA
* Corresponding author. University of Calgary, 1403 29 St NW, Calgary, Alberta, Canada T2N 2T9.
E-mail address: zahinoor@gmail.com

Psychiatr Clin N Am 36 (2013) 483–496
http://dx.doi.org/10.1016/j.psc.2013.08.010
0193-953X/13/$ – see front matter © 2013 Elsevier Inc. All rights reserved.
psych.theclinics.com

Abbreviations: Characterizing Late-Life Depression	
LLD	Late-life depression
MD	Major depression
MiND	Minor depression
HAM-D	Hamilton Depression Rating scale
GDS	Geriatric Depression Scale
SD	Subthreshold depression
BD	Bipolar depression
BAD	Bipolar affective disorder
OSA	Obstructive sleep apnea
PLMD	Periodic limb movement disorder
PSG	Polysomnography
REM	Rapid eye movement
REML	Rapid-eye-movement latencies
ECT	Electroconvulsive therapy
HRQOL	Health-related quality of life
CG	Complicated grief
MoCA	Montreal Cognitive Assessment

of aging. In most of the developed world, *old* is considered to be 65 years of age and older; although in parts of the developing world where life expectancies are much lower, this age may not be attained by many. Given the aging of the general population and access to medical care, there are now new categories being devised to accommodate the following: *young-old* for patients aged 65 to 75 years and *old-old* for patients older than 76 years. Thus, defining *old* is critically important to such fields as geriatric medicine and geriatric psychiatry. Services might only be provided to patients who fulfill certain age criteria, which may be considered somewhat arbitrary (ie, reaching 65 years of age and suddenly becoming eligible for geriatric services).

Another important distinction in geriatric psychiatry is between patients who are diagnosed with a disorder late in life and patients who experience a recurrence of their illness late in life. Research suggests that clinical symptoms and cause may differ considerably between these two groups. A differentiation is often made between patients who develop symptoms at a typical age and patients who develop symptoms late in life (late-life schizophrenia, late-life bipolar disorder, late-life depression [LLD]). The age criteria for late-onset disorders vary considerably. Late-onset schizophrenia and bipolar disorder, for example, are sometimes considered in patients aged 40 years and older, whereas late-onset depression is typically considered at 60 to 65 years of age. Because depression is a disorder that tends to occur across the lifespan, as opposed to having a peak age of onset, most studies have defined late-onset depression or depression in the elderly as being consistent with current definitions for *old* or *elderly* (aged 60 years, 65 years, and older). Similarly, most studies looking at treatment response in the elderly have used 60 to 65 years of age as a cutoff, both in the developed and developing world.[3]

HOW COMMON IS THE PROBLEM?

Although depression is common and clinically significant in late life, estimating its prevalence is challenging. Among other methodological issues, these challenges stem from variability in the definition of *late life* (as discussed earlier) as well as the measurement of depression. A review of the prevalence of depression in adults aged 65 years or older found a range from 0.9% to 42.0%, with clinically relevant depressive symptom cases in similar settings varying between 7.2% and 49.0%.[4]

A report on a series of Australian longitudinal studies on aging found that depression in older adults aged older than 60 years, stratified by decade, ranged from 1.1% to 34.4%.[5] When combining symptoms of major depression (MD) or minor depression with reported treatment of depression, the Aging, Demographics, and Memory Study found an overall depression prevalence of 11.19% in a cohort of Americans aged 71 years and older.[6] A systematic review and meta-analysis of 24 studies on the prevalence of depression in latest life (75 years and older) found that the prevalence of major depression ranged from 4.6% to 9.3% and that of depressive disorders from 4.5% to 37.4%. The pooled prevalence was 7.2% for major depression and 17.1% for depressive disorders.[7]

Fewer studies have estimated the incidence of LLD. A systematic review of LLD incidence in adults older than 70 years found that it varied considerably. MD was found to occur less often than minor depression (MinD), whereas clinically relevant depressive symptoms are at least as frequent as MinD. The incidence rate of MD was 0.2 to 14.1 per 100 person-years, and the incidence of clinically relevant depressive symptoms was 6.8 per 100 person-years.[8] Low incidence in the context of high prevalence implies a high degree of chronicity of depression in late life, once it occurs.

Confounding the prevalence and incidence estimates is the finding that depression has a variable course and trajectory in older adults. Early data from the Longitudinal Aging Study Amsterdam demonstrated that in older adults between 55 and 85 years of age, the prevalence of clinically significant depression was 14.9%, 2.02% of which met the criteria for major depressive disorder.[9] At the 6-year follow-up, 4 depressive trajectories were identified: short-lived symptoms, remissions, a fluctuating course, and a severe chronic course. For those with subthreshold depression (SD) at baseline, the risk of developing an affective disorder at 6 years was 27%, highlighting that depressive symptoms are not static but rather dynamic in late life.[10] A 12-year longitudinal study of 1260 community-dwelling adults in Pennsylvania aged 65 years and older identified 6 trajectories of depressive symptoms: 2 stable asymptomatic groups (starting with none or 1 symptom at baseline); a stable low-depressed group; an emerging-depressive-symptoms group; a remitting-depressive-symptoms group; and a persisting-depressive-symptoms group, which was associated with a higher medical burden and higher baseline scores.[11] A 10-year longitudinal study in 3922 Taiwanese adults aged 60 years and older identified 4 depressive trajectories (persistent low [41.8%], persistent mild [46.8%], late peak [4.2%], and high chronic [7.2%]) and an overall depression prevalence of 11.4%.[12] A 20-year longitudinal study of 7240 women aged 65 years or older identified 4 latent classes of depressive symptoms. These classes were minimal depressive symptoms (27.8%), persistently low depressive symptoms (54.0%), increasing depressive symptoms (14.8%), and persistently high depressive symptoms (3.4%). The risk factors for increasing depressive burden were baseline smoking, physical inactivity, small social network, physical impairment, myocardial infarction, diabetes, and obesity. Furthermore, survival to the oldest old was associated with increased depressive symptom burden.[13] Thus, although cross-sectional point prevalence estimates of depressive symptoms may vary, the identification of depression, whether subclinical or severe, is associated with a greater illness burden and poorer prognosis over time, requiring vigilance and ongoing assessment.

COMPLICATIONS AND DIFFERENCES IN SYMPTOMS BETWEEN YOUNG AND OLD PATIENTS WITH DEPRESSION

LLD in general is thought to have a worse prognosis, a more chronic course, and a higher relapse rate in general compared with patients who develop symptoms at a younger age.[14] It is also associated with higher levels of medical comorbidity, cognitive impairment, and mortality[15–17] and has a bidirectional relationship with frailty.[18] In addition, LLD may be associated with specific depressive syndromes, including vascular depression and depression-executive dysfunction syndrome.[19] With respect to cognition, there is substantial evidence that LLD has an adverse effect. Bhalla and colleagues[20] examined 56 patients aged 60 and older with LLD and compared them to 40 age- and education-matched nondepressed controls. Forty-five percent of the patients found to be cognitively impaired during the course of their depression continued to be cognitively impaired even when the depressive symptoms had remitted, 94% continued to be cognitively impaired 1 year later, and 23% of patients became cognitively impaired 1 year later despite being cognitively normal at baseline. Panza and colleagues[21] recently postulated that LLD may be on a continuum with mild cognitive impairment (MCI) and dementia. In a comprehensive review of previous studies, however, they found no evidence that depression led to an increased incidence of MCI or hastened conversion from MCI to frank dementia, although depressive symptoms in MCI do increase conversion rates to dementia.[22] Li and colleagues[23] followed a large sample of patients in the community aged 65 and older without dementia and discovered that early life depression had no impact on the future development of dementia, whereas LLD correlated with an increased risk of dementia of 1.46 (adjusted hazard ratio), suggesting LLD may perhaps be an early manifestation of dementia.

In addition to the medical complications, the symptomatic phenomenology may differ between old and young patients. This difference may reflect both generational issues as well as the realities of declining health. Older patients may be much more reluctant to express feeling sad and much more likely to focus on somatic issues.[24] In a recent meta-analysis, Hegeman and colleagues[25] looked at studies comparing the phenomenology of depression in older and younger patients. Patients had to meet the criteria for depression according to standardized criteria (*Diagnostic and Statistical Manual of Mental Disorders* [DSM], Research Diagnostic Criteria, *International Classification of Diseases*) and include a comparison of individual subscores of the Hamilton Depression Rating scale (HAM-D). Eleven studies were included, and older patients relative to younger patients were found to have more agitation, hypochondriasis, somatic preoccupation (including gastrointestinal), less guilt, and loss of sexual interest.[25] The meta-analysis surprisingly showed no difference in the HAM-D criteria of loss of insight, work, and activity and psychomotor retardation between early and late-onset patients. There was also no difference in depressed mood, which was in contrast to what has been found in previous studies.[24,26,27] Studies have also shown that older patients with MD when compared with younger patients are more likely to endorse the so-called cognitive symptoms of depression, including hopelessness, worthlessness, and guilt.[28] However, not all studies to date have shown differences in symptom profiles between the old and young.[29–34]

The overlap between apathy and depression is another area of controversy, given that patients with apathy may be wrongly diagnosed with depression, leading to further confusion around phenomenology.[35,36] Mehta and colleagues[37] looked at depressive symptoms in a cohort of young-old (less than 80 years of age) and old-old (greater than 80 years of age) patients and discovered in the young-old subgroup that resilience, apathy, and disability contributed equally to the variance in the Geriatric Depression Scale (GDS) scores, whereas apathy was the greatest contributor in old-old patients. Examining how to account for physical symptoms in older patients with depression has led to the evolution of different approaches, including the inclusive approach (all symptoms are included regardless of type), the exclusive approach (physical symptoms are excluded), the etiologic approach (only symptoms not caused by physical disease are included), and the substitutive approach (physical symptoms are replaced by nonsomatic alternatives). Different approaches result in a different appreciation of depression in this patient population.

SUBSYNDROMAL DEPRESSION

Subsyndromal and SD are clinical symptoms of depression of insufficient severity to meet the diagnostic criteria for MD. This distinction can be somewhat artificial as evidenced by a Finnish study that demonstrated even minor wording changes in a highly structured rating instrument resulted in different prevalence rates of depression in 5993 patients aged 15 to 75 years.[38] Furthermore, DSM criteria may or may not accurately diagnose major depression in the elderly, resulting in a greater spillover into the subthreshold category.[39,40] Nonetheless, SD is associated with adverse functional outcomes, increased risk for incident Axis I and II psychopathology, increased psychosocial disability, and economic and societal cost.[41] The Berlin Aging Study found that in adults 70 years or older, SD can be characterized in 2 ways: as a quantitatively minor variant of depression (ie, a depressionlike state with fewer symptoms) or as qualitatively different from major depression with fewer suicidal thoughts or feelings of guilt or worthlessness.[42] In a primary care population of adults aged 65 years or older, SD with a history of MD increased the risk of developing a depressive diagnosis in the subsequent 3 months.[43] Another primary care study of adults aged 65 years and older demonstrated that patients with SD had poorer outcomes at 1 year in terms of psychiatric symptoms and functional status, often not significantly different than MD or MinD.[44] A Swedish cohort of primary care patients aged 60 years or older described 3 courses of SD (remitting, stable, and fluctuating), highlighting the importance of identifying SD and following with longitudinal assessments.[45] Finally, a review of SD showed that in addition to being 2 to 3 times more prevalent than MD in older adults, 8% to 10% of older adults with SD developed MD per year. Although the course of SD was more favorable than MD, it was found to be far from benign, with only 27% remitting to nondepressed status after 1 year.[46] Clearly further research is required into SD, especially with respect to treatment and outcomes.

BIPOLAR DEPRESSION IN THE ELDERLY

It is estimated that as many as 10% of patients diagnosed with unipolar depression at some point in their lives may have bipolar depression (BD).[47] When this definition is broadened to include patients within the bipolar spectrum or patients who experience some form of mood elevation, the rates increase to as much as 50%.[48,49] To date, there have been no large-scale multicentered studies examining the prevalence or clinical correlates of bipolar affective disorder (BAD) in the elderly, let alone BD.[50] However, a review of the data from several recent community surveys both in the United States[51] and Europe[52] suggests a lifetime prevalence of 1% for bipolar type I and 1.2% for bipolar type II. There is a suggestion that although unipolar depression increases in prevalence with age, BD starts when patients are much younger, typically by the third decade.[53] This finding is consistent with a recent review by Depp and Jeste,[50] which showed the prevalence of BAD decreases significantly with age based on a review of community surveys, similar to depression and schizophrenia. The Epidemiologic Catchment Area (ECA) survey confirms a 1-year prevalence of 0.1% among adults older than 65 years of age, down from 1.4% for young adults (18–44 years) and 0.4% for middle-aged adults (45–64 years). Other community-based surveys have quoted similar percentages, including 0.5% based on a community survey conducted by Hirschfeld and colleagues (2003),[54] 0.08% based on a telephone survey,[3] and 0.25% based on an administrative database survey. Inpatient psychiatry samples for BD are likely misleading because they focus primarily on mania. In any case, estimates range from 4.7%[55] to 18.5%.[56] Outpatient clinic estimates for BAD in general range from 2%[57] to 8%.[58] It is estimated that 90% of patients with BAD will develop symptoms by the age of 50 years,[59] with only 10% qualifying for a diagnosis of late-onset disease. Prevalence rates in institutionalized settings, such as nursing homes[60] and inpatient units,[50] are estimated to be considerably higher. One of the few studies to look specifically at the prevalence of late-life BD was conducted by Takeshima and colleagues.[61] This study looked retrospectively at a subset of patients older than 60 years who were admitted to the hospital with a diagnosis of major depressive disorder (MDD). A total of 36.8% of patients were diagnosed with BAD, whereas 63.2% were diagnosed with a MDD, and 81.3% of the BAD sample were estimated to have bipolar type II along with 29.9% of the MDD sample. In mixed-age cohorts, the prevalence rate of bipolar type II associated with a MDD is estimated to be about 50%.[62,63] There is a general consensus that the subtype of BAD most commonly associated with depression, bipolar type II, is underdiagnosed.[54,63]

Apart from formal diagnostic criteria, studies have attempted to compare older patients with BD to other diagnostic subgroups in terms of their functional and psychiatric status. Compared with patients with schizophrenia, older patients with BD have been found to have more depressive symptoms, similar cognitive functioning, and fewer positive/negative symptoms.[64] Compared with older patients with unipolar depression, older patients with BD have been found to have worse functional status, more positive symptoms, and similar cognitive status.[65] Thus, older patients with BAD have a functional/psychiatric status that is in between schizophrenia and unipolar depression. In terms of common comorbidities, studies have recently shown that late-life BAD is commonly comorbid with alcohol abuse, panic attacks, generalized anxiety disorder, and dysthymia.[66]

SLEEP, QUALITY OF LIFE, AND SUICIDE

Sleep problems, including both insomnia and hypersomnia, are among the most common symptoms of MD at any age, and aging itself is associated with an increasing prevalence of insomnia.[67] However, sleep problems in LLD are particularly vexing and complicated. Apart from the misery that accompanies being awake in the middle of the night, unresolved symptoms of insomnia are a risk factor for first episodes of depression[68] and also for depressive relapse in the elderly.[69] Investigations are underway to clarify whether treatment of insomnia can either prevent first lifetime episodes of MD or reduce the risk of relapse.

Insomnia symptom profiles in depressed patients are shaped by aging. Early morning awakening is an insomnia symptom most often seen in older depressed patients as opposed to younger depressed patients.[70] This fact may be related to an age-dependent phase advance in the entire rest-activity cycle. Starting as early as the third decade, the clock time for the sleeping period becomes earlier and earlier, and this process continues through at least the seventh decade. The authors have found that in depressed patients with insomnia, the midpoint of the sleep period creeps an average of 4 minutes earlier for each year of age.[71] By implication, the treatment planning for the sleep problems in LLD should assume that the behavioral targets for most older patients should include an earlier bedtime and an earlier rising time than would be targeted in younger depressed patients.

Insomnia symptoms in LLD can be complicated by the lack of structure that comes with retirement.[72] Many older people look forward to retirement as a time when they can tailor their sleep habits as they see fit, without respect to a work schedule. This attitude can lead to laxity in sleeping habits, which in turn results in erratic wake-up times in the morning and excessive time in bed, both of which can aggravate broken sleep. Patients with insomnia in the context of LLD should be encouraged to have the same rising time 7 days per week and to spend no more than 8 hours in bed.

The prevalence of primary sleep disorders, such as obstructive sleep apnea (OSA) and restless leg syndrome/periodic limb movement disorder (PLMD), increases with age; the cardinal symptoms of these disorders in young adults may be absent in the elderly.[73] Further, occult OSA and PLMD have a combined prevalence of about 15% in depressed patients who were otherwise not suspected of having a primary sleep disorder.[74] Failure to identify primary sleep disorders could hinder the treatment of LLD; some investigators, but not others,[75] have shown that treatment of OSA reduces at least some symptoms of MD.[76,77]

Still, polysomnography (PSG) should be used only selectively in patients with LLD, perhaps reserved for patients with obvious signs and symptoms of a primary sleep disorder or whose sleep symptoms fail to respond to standard treatment. Outside of the clinical setting, PSG has been used as a research tool and shows predictable differences in the progression of sleep stages in patients with MD versus normal controls. Patients with MD have a shorter latency between sleep onset and the onset of rapid-eye-movement (REM) sleep, and this finding is particularly pronounced in LLD.[70] REM latencies (REML) are generally 90 to 100 minutes in healthy adults but may be as short as 20 to 60 minutes in older people with depression. REM sleep abnormalities have been linked to a need for biologic therapies, such as pharmacotherapy or electroconvulsive therapy (ECT),[78] and a poorer response to psychotherapy alone.[79,80] Short REML has also been linked to suicide risk.[81]

Insomnia has a negative impact on health-related quality of life (HRQOL) in patients with depression.[82] Poor HRQOL is a defining feature of MD; HRQOL is rated lower by patients with depression versus patients with other common ambulatory health problems, such as hypertension.[83] The overall negative impact of depression on HRQOL is proportional to the intensity of depressive symptoms.[84] However, the phenotype of poor HRQOL is different in older depressed patients as contrasted with younger depressed patients. Younger depressed patients complain of greater negative impact of the illness on their relationships, whereas older depressed patients describe comparatively greater negative impact of the illness on their ability to carry out basic chores of living and housekeeping.[85] A failure to perform basic functions, such as food shopping, meal preparation, and housekeeping, may represent an urgent threat to the independence of an older depressed person who is living alone. Perhaps for this reason, ECT is offered more often to older depressed patients as opposed to younger depressed patients.[85]

Suicidal behavior and suicide death are the greatest concern in the care of patients with LLD. A serious suicide attempt, such as a self-inflicted gunshot wound, or even suicide death may occasionally be the initial presentation of LLD. Suicide death increases across the life cycle but especially for older Caucasian men.[86] The increase in suicide rates with age may be related to the accumulation of chronic medical conditions and the isolation that accompanies divorce or widowhood. Insomnia is an independent risk factor for suicidal ideation for adults[87,88] and suicide death in the elderly.[89,90] Whether the treatment of insomnia can mitigate the suicide risk in LLD is unknown. As with patients of all ages, worsening suicidal ideation may indicate hospitalization and perhaps the need for ECT.[91,92]

RELATIONSHIP BETWEEN GRIEF AND DEPRESSION

Grief can be a confounding factor in the understanding of LLD, especially given the higher likelihood of bereavement with advancing age. Bereavement refers to the state of having lost someone emotionally important, and grief is an instinctual response to bereavement that includes a person's thoughts, feelings, and behaviors.[93] Fifteen percent of grievers can face complications, such as MD; this can be comorbid or confounded by complicated grief (CG), which occurs in 10% to 20%.[94] Latent class analysis of depressive symptoms in participants from the Cache County Study identified 3 depressive subgroups: significantly depressed (62%); a group with low probability of any symptoms other than sadness (21%); and a group with primarily psychomotor changes, sleep symptoms, and fatigue (17%). The first group was akin to clinical or MD and most likely to be treated with antidepressants and yet had the greatest likelihood of recently being bereaved.[95] There are distinctions between bereavement-related depression and CG, which may help distinguish the two. Factor analysis has identified loneliness as loading onto depression versus lack of acceptance of the death as loading onto CG.[96] Grief does not resolve as quickly as depression,[97] even when treated with antidepressants,[98] and may require further grief-specific therapies.[94] Thus, although grief and depression can look similar, and even overlap, they have different trajectories and treatments.

SUMMARY

LLD is common and associated with significant medical and psychiatric comorbidity. Depressive symptoms in late life are not stable and can be associated with different trajectories over time. Thus, subsyndromal depression is an important and underappreciated state and should be followed over time. There are significant comorbidities with LLD, including medical illness, frailty, sleep disturbance, grief, and cognitive impairment. Greater vigilance is required for all comorbidities in patients with LLD.

CLINICAL VIGNETTE: BEREAVEMENT WITH PHYSICAL COMORBIDITIES

A 76-year-old woman presents to the clinic in referral from her family doctor for the assessment and management of bereavement. Formerly a physiotherapist and very active mother of 3, she has become listless, frail, and sad in the wake of her husband's death, which was sudden, 3 months ago. She has a history of hypertension and a deep vein thrombosis and is on medications for this. She has been less consistent in taking her medications, and her blood pressure has been labile. Most recently she slipped in the kitchen, bruised her hip, and sustained a Colles fracture. Her recovery from this has been slower than expected. Her daughter triggered the referral after telling the family doctor that the patient had expressed some thoughts of wanting to die in addition to sadness, loneliness, weight loss, and terminal insomnia. On obtaining further history from another daughter, it turns out she has likely had some decline in function for 6 months prior to her husband's death as evidenced by increased reliance on him for social activity and subtle anxiety, but little was thought of it at the time. These symptoms have become more evident of late to the extent that her daughter brought her to live in her home. She was tearful in the office and had feelings of guilt and hopelessness. Her GDS-15 score was 9; she endorsed multiple symptoms, both psychological and somatic. Her Montreal Cognitive Assessment (MoCA) score at the time was 23 out of 30, losing points for trail making, attention, and short-term memory. An antidepressant was started, and she was encouraged to attend a day program. After 6 weeks, her family stated that she looked brighter and was sleeping longer, although the patient did not appreciate this. At 12 weeks, she was significantly better with only residual symptoms and was resuming activity and seeing more of her friends. She was future oriented and had no thoughts of dying. Although she wanted to return to her home, her daughter was apprehensive still because she felt that despite significant improvements, her mother had not fully returned to previous levels of functioning. Her repeat MoCA score was 25 out of 30, with slightly better short-term memory but no other changes in domain scores.

This case highlights the difficulties in distinguishing grief from depression and the importance of obtaining premorbid levels of functioning. Although initially looking like the aftermath of bereavement, history and phenomenology supported a diagnosis of MD, late onset, which responded well to antidepressant treatment. Notwithstanding the improvements, some subtle cognitive deficits remained, even after symptom remission. It was decided to follow her up from a cognitive status, the results of which are still pending.

REFERENCES

1. Rowe JW, Kahn RL. Human aging: usual and successful. Science 1987; 237(4811):143–9.
2. Cohen GD. Historical lessons to watch your assumptions about aging: relevance to the role of International Psychogeriatrics. Int Psychogeriatr 2009; 21(3):425–9.
3. Kessler RC, Andrews G, Mroczek D. The World Health Organization Composite International Diagnostic Interview Short-Form (CIDI-SF). Int J Methods Psychiatr Res 1998;7(4):171–85.
4. Djernes JK. Prevalence and predictors of depression in populations of elderly: a review. Acta Psychiatr Scand 2006;113(5):372–87.
5. Burns RA, Butterworth P, Windsor TD, et al. Deriving prevalence estimates of depressive symptoms throughout middle and old age in those living in the community. Int Psychogeriatr 2012;24(3):503–11.
6. Steffens DC, Fisher GG, Langa KM, et al. Prevalence of depression among older Americans: the Aging, Demographics and Memory Study. Int Psychogeriatr 2009;21(5):879–88.
7. Luppa M, Sikorski C, Luck T, et al. Age- and gender-specific prevalence of depression in latest-life–systematic review and meta-analysis. J Affect Disord 2012;136(3):212–21.
8. Buchtemann D, Luppa M, Bramesfeld A, et al. Incidence of late-life depression: a systematic review. J Affect Disord 2012;142(1–3):172–9.
9. Beekman AT, Deeg DJ, van Tilburg T, et al. Major and minor depression in later life: a study of prevalence and risk factors. J Affect Disord 1995;36(1–2):65–75.
10. Beekman AT, Geerlings SW, Deeg DJ, et al. The natural history of late-life depression: a 6-year prospective study in the community. Arch Gen Psychiatry 2002;59(7):605–11.
11. Andreescu C, Chang CC, Mulsant BH, et al. Twelve-year depressive symptom trajectories and their predictors in a community sample of older adults. Int Psychogeriatr 2008;20(2):221–36.
12. Kuo SY, Lin KM, Chen CY, et al. Depression trajectories and obesity among the elderly in Taiwan. Psychol Med 2011;41(8):1665–76.
13. Byers AL, Vittinghoff E, Lui LY, et al. Twenty-year depressive trajectories among older women. Arch Gen Psychiatry 2012;69(10):1073–9.
14. Mitchell AJ, Subramaniam H. Prognosis of depression in old age compared to middle age: a systematic review of comparative studies. Am J Psychiatry 2005;162(9):1588–601.
15. Penninx BWJH, Beekman ATF, Bandinelli S, et al. Late-life depressive symptoms are associated with both hyperactivity and hypoactivity of the hypothalamo-pituitary-adrenal axis. Am J Geriatr Psychiatry 2007;15(6):522.

16. Penninx BWJH, Guralnik JM, Mendes de Leon CF, et al. Cardiovascular events and mortality in newly and chronically depressed persons > 70 years of age. Am J Cardiol 1998;81(8):988–94.

17. Baldwin RC, Gallagley A, Gourlay M, et al. Prognosis of late life depression: a three-year cohort study of outcome and potential predictors. Int J Geriatr Psychiatry 2006;21(1):57–63.

18. Mezuk B, Edwards L, Lohman M, et al. Depression and frailty in later life: a synthetic review. Int J Geriatr Psychiatry 2012;27(9):879–92.

19. Alexopoulos GS, Katz IR, Bruce ML, et al. Remission in depressed geriatric primary care patients: a report from the PROSPECT study. Am J Psychiatry 2005; 162(4):718.

20. Bhalla RK, Butters MA, Mulsant BH, et al. Persistence of neuropsychologic deficits in the remitted state of late-life depression. Am J Geriatr Psychiatry 2006; 14(5):419–27.

21. Panza F, Frisardi V, Capurso C, et al. Late-life depression, mild cognitive impairment, and dementia: possible continuum? Am J Geriatr Psychiatry 2010; 18(2):98.

22. Modrego PJ, Ferrandez J. Depression in patients with mild cognitive impairment increases the risk of developing dementia of Alzheimer type: a prospective cohort study. Arch Neurol 2004;61(8):1290–3.

23. Li G, Wang LY, Shofer JB, et al. Temporal relationship between depression and dementia: findings from a large community-based 15-year follow-up study. Arch Gen Psychiatry 2011;68(9):970.

24. Thomas A. Oxford textbook of old age psychiatry. New York: Oxford University Press; 2008.

25. Hegeman J, Kok R, van der Mast R, et al. Phenomenology of depression in older compared with younger adults: meta-analysis. Br J Psychiatry 2012;200(4): 275–81.

26. Gatz M, Hurwicz ML. Are old people more depressed? Cross-sectional data on Center for Epidemiological Studies Depression Scale factors. Psychol Aging 1990;5(2):284.

27. Gurland BJ. The comparative frequency of depression in various adult age groups. J Gerontol 1976;31(3):283–92.

28. Gallo JJ, Anthony JC, Muthen BO. Age differences in the symptoms of depression: a latent trait analysis. J Gerontol 1994;49(6):P251–64.

29. Musetti L, Perugi G, Soriani A, et al. Depression before and after age 65. A reexamination. Br J Psychiatry 1989;155(3):330–6.

30. Weissman MM. The myth of involutional melancholia. JAMA 1979;242(8):742–4.

31. Wesner RB, Winokur G. An archival study of depression before and after age 55. J Geriatr Psychiatry Neurol 1988;1(4):220–5.

32. Blazer D, Hughes DC, George LK. The epidemiology of depression in an elderly community population. Gerontologist 1987;27(3):281–7.

33. Corruble E, Gorwood P, Falissard B. Association between age of onset and symptom profiles of late-life depression. Acta Psychiatr Scand 2008;118(5):389–94.

34. Gallagher D, Mhaolain AN, Greene E, et al. Late life depression: a comparison of risk factors and symptoms according to age of onset in community dwelling older adults. Int J Geriatr Psychiatry 2010;25(10):981–7.

35. Newson RS, Hek K, Luijendijk HJ, et al. Atherosclerosis and incident depression in late life. Arch Gen Psychiatry 2010;67(11):1144.

36. Van der Mast R, Vinkers D, Stek M, et al. Vascular disease and apathy in old age. The Leiden 85-plus Study. Int J Geriatr Psychiatry 2007;23(3):266–71.

37. Mehta M, Whyte E, Lenze E, et al. Depressive symptoms in late life: associations with apathy, resilience and disability vary between young-old and old-old. Int J Geriatr Psychiatry 2008;23(3):238–43.
38. Karlsson L, Marttunen M, Karlsson H, et al. Minor change in the diagnostic threshold leads into major alteration in the prevalence estimate of depression. J Affect Disord 2010;122(1–2):96–101.
39. Cherubini A, Nistico G, Rozzini R, et al. Subthreshold depression in older subjects: an unmet therapeutic need. J Nutr Health Aging 2012;16(10):909–13.
40. Anderson TM, Slade T, Andrews G, et al. DSM-IV major depressive episode in the elderly: the relationship between the number and the type of depressive symptoms and impairment. J Affect Disord 2009;117(1–2):55–62.
41. Pietrzak RH, Kinley J, Afifi TO, et al. Subsyndromal depression in the United States: prevalence, course, and risk for incident psychiatric outcomes. Psychol Med 2012;43(7):1–14.
42. Geiselmann B, Bauer M. Subthreshold depression in the elderly: qualitative or quantitative distinction? Compr Psychiatry 2000;41(2 Suppl 1):32–8.
43. Chopra MP, Zubritsky C, Knott K, et al. Importance of subsyndromal symptoms of depression in elderly patients. Am J Geriatr Psychiatry 2005;13(7):597–606.
44. Grabovich A, Lu N, Tang W, et al. Outcomes of subsyndromal depression in older primary care patients. Am J Geriatr Psychiatry 2010;18(3):227–35.
45. Magnil M, Janmarker L, Gunnarsson R, et al. Course, risk factors, and prognostic factors in elderly primary care patients with mild depression: a two-year observational study. Scand J Prim Health Care 2013;31(1):20–5.
46. Meeks TW, Vahia IV, Lavretsky H, et al. A tune in "a minor" can "b major": a review of epidemiology, illness course, and public health implications of subthreshold depression in older adults. J Affect Disord 2011;129(1–3):126–42.
47. Goodwin GM, Anderson I, Arango C, et al. ECNP consensus meeting. Bipolar depression. Nice, March 2007. Eur Neuropsychopharmacol 2008;18(7):535–49.
48. Angst J, Gamma A, Benazzi F, et al. Toward a re-definition of subthreshold bipolarity: epidemiology and proposed criteria for bipolar-II, minor bipolar disorders and hypomania. J Affect Disord 2003;73(1–2):133–46.
49. Cassano GB, Rucci P, Frank E, et al. The mood spectrum in unipolar and bipolar disorder: arguments for a unitary approach. Am J Psychiatry 2004;161(7):1264–9.
50. Depp CA, Jeste DV. Bipolar disorder in older adults: a critical review. Bipolar Disord 2004;6(5):343–67.
51. Merikangas KR, Akiskal HS, Angst J, et al. Lifetime and 12-month prevalence of bipolar spectrum disorder in the National Comorbidity Survey replication. Arch Gen Psychiatry 2007;64(5):543.
52. Pini S, de Queiroz V, Pagnin D, et al. Prevalence and burden of bipolar disorders in European countries. Eur Neuropsychopharmacol 2005;15(4):425–34.
53. Wittchen HU, Muehlig S, Pezawas L. Natural course and burden of bipolar disorders. Int J Neuropsychopharmacol 2003;6(2):145–54.
54. Hirschfeld R, Calabrese JR, Weissman MM, et al. Screening for bipolar disorder in the community. J Clin Psychiatry 2003;64(1):53.
55. Yassa R, Nair V, Nastase C, et al. Prevalence of bipolar disorder in a psychogeriatric population. J Affect Disord 1988;14(3):197–201.
56. Moak GS. Characteristics of demented and nondemented geriatric admissions to a state hospital. Hosp Community Psychiatry 1990;41:799–801.
57. Speer DC. Differences in social resources and treatment history among diagnostic groups of older adults. Hosp Community Psychiatry 1992;43(3):270–4.

58. Molinari VA, Chacko RC, Rosenberg SD. Bipolar disorder in the elderly. J Psychiatr Treat Eval 1983;5(4):325–30.
59. Hirschfeld RMA, Lewis L, Vornik LA. Perceptions and impact of bipolar disorder: how far have we really come? Results of the National Depressive and Manic-Depressive Association 2000 survey of individuals with bipolar disorder. J Clin Psychiatry 2003;64(2):161–74.
60. Koenig HG, Blazer DG. Epidemiology of geriatric affective disorders. Clin Geriatr Med 1992;8(2):235.
61. Takeshima M, Kurata K. Late-life bipolar depression due to the soft form of bipolar disorder compared to unipolar depression: an inpatient chart review study. J Affect Disord 2010;123(1):64–70.
62. Benazzi F. Prevalence of bipolar II disorder in outpatient depression: a 203-case study in private practice. J Affect Disord 1997;43(2):163–6.
63. Hantouche EG, Akiskal HS, Lancrenon S, et al. Systematic clinical methodology for validating bipolar-II disorder: data in mid-stream from a French national multi-site study (EPIDEP). J Affect Disord 1998;50(2–3):163.
64. Bartels SJ, Mueser KT, Miles KM. A comparative study of elderly patients with schizophrenia and bipolar disorder in nursing homes and the community. Schizophr Res 1997;27(2):181–90.
65. Bartels SJ, Forester B, Miles KM, et al. Mental health service use by elderly patients with bipolar disorder and unipolar major depression. Am J Geriatr Psychiatry 2000;8(2):160–6.
66. Goldstein BI, Herrmann N, Shulman KI. Comorbidity in bipolar disorder among the elderly: results from an epidemiological community sample. Am J Psychiatry 2006;163(2):319–21.
67. Ancoli-Israel S, Roth T. Characteristics of insomnia in the United States: results of the 1991 National Sleep Foundation Survey. I. Sleep 1999;22(Suppl 2):S347–53.
68. Ford DE, Kamerow DB. Epidemiologic study of sleep disturbances and psychiatric disorders. An opportunity for prevention? JAMA 1989;262(11):1479–84.
69. Reynolds CF 3rd, Frank E, Houck PR, et al. Which elderly patients with remitted depression remain well with continued interpersonal psychotherapy after discontinuation of antidepressant medication? Am J Psychiatry 1997;154(7):958–62.
70. Gillin JC, Duncan WC, Murphy DL, et al. Age-related changes in sleep in depressed and normal subjects. Psychiatry Res 1981;4(1):73–8.
71. McCall WV, Gonzales C, Shannon W. Age-related effects on circadian phase in the sleep of depressed insomniacs, in Association of Professional Sleep Societies. Boston: 2012.
72. Ohayon MM, Zulley J, Guilleminault C, et al. How age and daytime activities are related to insomnia in the general population: consequences for older people. J Am Geriatr Soc 2001;49(4):360–6.
73. Stradling JR, Davies RJ. Sleep. 1: obstructive sleep apnoea/hypopnoea syndrome: definitions, epidemiology, and natural history. Thorax 2004;59(1):73–8.
74. McCall WV, Kimball J, Boggs N, et al. Prevalence and prediction of primary sleep disorders in a clinical trial of depressed patients with insomnia. J Clin Sleep Med 2009;5(5):454–8.
75. Lee IS, Bardwell W, Ancoli-Israel S, et al. Effect of three weeks of continuous positive airway pressure treatment on mood in patients with obstructive sleep apnoea: a randomized placebo-controlled study. Sleep Med 2012;13(2):161–6.

76. El-Sherbini AM, Bediwy AS, El-Mitwalli A. Association between obstructive sleep apnea (OSA) and depression and the effect of continuous positive airway pressure (CPAP) treatment. Neuropsychiatr Dis Treat 2011;7:715–21.

77. Habukawa M, Uchimura N, Kakuma T, et al. Effect of CPAP treatment on residual depressive symptoms in patients with major depression and coexisting sleep apnea: contribution of daytime sleepiness to residual depressive symptoms. Sleep Med 2010;11(6):552–7.

78. Coffey CE, McCall WV, Hoelscher TJ, et al. Effects of ECT on polysomnographic sleep: a prospective investigation. Convuls Ther 1988;4(4):269–79.

79. Thase ME, Buysse DJ, Frank E, et al. Which depressed patients will respond to interpersonal psychotherapy? The role of abnormal EEG sleep profiles. Am J Psychiatry 1997;154(4):502–9.

80. Thase ME, Simons AD, Reynolds CF 3rd. Abnormal electroencephalographic sleep profiles in major depression: association with response to cognitive behavior therapy. Arch Gen Psychiatry 1996;53(2):99–108.

81. Agargun MY, Cartwright R. REM sleep, dream variables and suicidality in depressed patients. Psychiatry Res 2003;119(1–2):33–9.

82. McCall WV, Reboussin BA, Cohen W. Subjective measurement of insomnia and quality of life in depressed inpatients. J Sleep Res 2000;9(1):43–8.

83. Wells KB, Stewart A, Hays RD, et al. The functioning and well-being of depressed patients. Results from the Medical Outcomes Study. JAMA 1989; 262(7):914–9.

84. McCall WV, Cohen W, Reboussin B, et al. Effects of mood and age on quality of life in depressed inpatients. J Affect Disord 1999;55(2–3):107–14.

85. McCall WV, Cohen W, Reboussin B, et al. Pretreatment differences in specific symptoms and quality of life among depressed inpatients who do and do not receive electroconvulsive therapy: a hypothesis regarding why the elderly are more likely to receive ECT. J ECT 1999;15(3):193–201.

86. Hawton K, van Heeringen K. Suicide. Lancet 2009;373(9672):1372–81.

87. McCall WV. Insomnia is a risk factor for suicide-what are the next steps? Sleep 2011;34(9):1149–50.

88. McCall WV, Blocker JN, D'Agostino R Jr, et al. Insomnia severity is an indicator of suicidal ideation during a depression clinical trial. Sleep Med 2010;11(9): 822–7.

89. Fujino Y, Mizoue T, Tokui N, et al. Prospective cohort study of stress, life satisfaction, self-rated health, insomnia, and suicide death in Japan. Suicide Life Threat Behav 2005;35(2):227–37.

90. Turvey CL, Conwell Y, Jones MP, et al. Risk factors for late-life suicide: a prospective, community-based study. Am J Geriatr Psychiatry 2002;10(4):398–406.

91. McCall WV. What does Star*D tell us about ECT? J ECT 2007;23(1):1–2.

92. Kellner CH, Fink M, Knapp R, et al. Relief of expressed suicidal intent by ECT: a consortium for research in ECT study. Am J Psychiatry 2005;162(5):977–82.

93. Miller MD. Complicated grief in late life. Dialogues Clin Neurosci 2012;14(2): 195–202.

94. Shear K, Frank E, Houck PR, et al. Treatment of complicated grief: a randomized controlled trial. JAMA 2005;293(21):2601–8.

95. Lee CT, Leoutsakos JM, Lyketsos CG, et al. Latent class-derived subgroups of depressive symptoms in a community sample of older adults: the Cache County Study. Int J Geriatr Psychiatry 2012;27(10):1061–9.

96. Lichtenthal WG, Cruess DG, Prigerson HG. A case for establishing complicated grief as a distinct mental disorder in DSM-V. Clin Psychol Rev 2004;24(6):637–62.

97. Pasternak RE, Reynolds CF, Frank E, et al. The temporal course of depressive symptoms and grief intensity in late-life spousal bereavement. Depression 1993;1:45–9.
98. Pasternak RE, Reynolds CF 3rd, Schlernitzauer M, et al. Acute open-trial nortriptyline therapy of bereavement-related depression in late life. J Clin Psychiatry 1991;52(7):307–10.

What Are the Causes of Late-Life Depression?

Rehan Aziz, MD[a,b,c],*, David C. Steffens, MD, MHS[c]

KEYWORDS

- Late life • Geriatric • Depression • Psychological • Social factors in late life

KEY POINTS

- Depressive symptoms in elders have been associated with impairment similar to that of major depressive disorder.
- Depressive disorders in the geriatric age range are found in 3.0% to 4.5% of the population.
- Late-onset depression has been prominently linked to cerebrovascular compromise.
- Depression likely serves as both a risk factor and potentially an early sign of dementia.
- The most significant psychosocial factors leading to depression are bereavement; perceived social support; neuroticism; personality disorders; loneliness; disability; total number of life events; total number of daily hassles; and impaired social support, including lack of a confidante.

OVERVIEW

The rapid increase in the numbers of older adults worldwide makes a focus on mental disorders and aging both timely and imperative. According to the 2010 census, in the United States, there were 40.3 million adults aged 65 years and older. This number represented an increase of 5.3 million over the 2000 census. Between 2000 and 2010, the number of elders increased at a faster rate (15.1%) than the total US population (9.7%).[1] These numbers are projected to continue to diverge, and the disparity between age groups will widen further as a consequence. By 2050, an estimated 20.2% of the population will be 65 years of age and older.[2]

Financial Disclosures: R. Aziz has nothing to disclose. D.C. Steffens has received grant support from the National Institutes of Health (NIH) and royalties from the American Psychiatric Association (APA) for textbooks related to geriatric psychiatry.

[a] Department of Psychiatry, Institute of Living, Hartford Hospital, 200 Retreat Avenue, Hartford, CT 06106, USA; [b] Department of Psychiatry, Yale University School of Medicine, 300 George Street, Suite 901, New Haven, CT 06511, USA; [c] Department of Psychiatry, University of Connecticut Health Center, Building L, MC 1410, 263 Farmington Avenue, Farmington, CT 06030, USA
* Corresponding author. Department of Psychiatry, Institute of Living, Hartford Hospital, 200 Retreat Avenue, Hartford, CT 06106.
E-mail address: Rehan.Aziz@hhchealth.org

Psychiatr Clin N Am 36 (2013) 497–516
http://dx.doi.org/10.1016/j.psc.2013.08.001
0193-953X/13/$ – see front matter © 2013 Elsevier Inc. All rights reserved.

Abbreviations: Description of Depression in Later Life	
MMSE	Mini-Mental State Examination
MDD	Major depressive disorder
EOD	Early onset depression
LOD	Late-onset depression
DSM-IV-TR	*Diagnostic and Statistical Manual of Mental Disorders* (Fourth Edition, Text Revision)
ECA	Epidemiologic Catchment Area
IOM	Institute of Medicine
GDS	Geriatric Depression Scale
MTHFR	Methyltetrahydrofolate reductase
CBS	Cystathionine beta-synthetase
CADASIL	Cerebral autosomal dominant arteriopathy with subcortical infarcts and leukoencephalopathy
ACC	Anterior cingulate cortex
OFC	Orbitofrontal cortex
rCFB	Regional cerebral blood flow
DLPFC	Dorsolateral prefrontal cortex
WMH	White matter hyperintensities

CLINICAL VIGNETTE: ELDERLY WOMAN WITH DEPRESSION

Ms S was a 73-year-old widowed white woman with a past psychiatric history significant for major depressive disorder (MDD), recurrent, severe without psychotic features, and a past medical history significant for hypertension, hypercholesterolemia, and a cerebrovascular accident who was seen, at the urging of her daughters, for evaluation of depression in a geriatric psychiatry outpatient clinic. Over the previous 2 months, Ms S had become increasingly depressed. She reported frequent crying spells, poor sleep quality, difficulty falling asleep, frequent nighttime awakenings, low energy, and limited concentration. She denied psychotic symptoms or suicidal ideation. She was taking paroxetine 20 mg/d.

Ms S had a history of depression dating back approximately 15 years. Her depression had occurred in the context of significant financial distress, her husband's passing, and a left internal capsule lacunar infarct. During the course of that initial episode, she had failed to respond to several medications and ultimately received a course of 14 sessions of electroconvulsive therapy to which she had responded well. Over the years, she had also been trialed on sertraline and citalopram for recurrent, though less severe, bouts of depression.

A mental status examination revealed a melancholy older woman with little spontaneous movement and moderate psychomotor retardation. Her speech pattern had high latency. She had a constricted affect and was sporadically tearful during the interview. She described her mood as low. There was no evidence of psychosis or suicidality. She scored 28 of 30 on the Mini-Mental State Examination (MMSE).

Ms S was started on extended-release venlafaxine. Her dose was gradually increased to 75 mg daily. Paroxetine was tapered off. At her next follow-up visit, Ms S reported no depressive symptoms.

At a follow-up visit 18 months later, her mood remained euthymic. However, during the session, Ms S had difficulty processing information. Her MMSE score was 21; she had errors regarding the year, the date, the day of the week, the month, the country, and the floor of the building; spelled the word WORLD in a convoluted manner (DLROE); recalled only one of 3 items; and had difficulty placing a sheet of paper on her lap. Ms S received a brain magnetic resonance imaging (MRI) (Fig. 1). This MRI was compared to an earlier MRI, which had already established the presence of cerebrovascular disease. Ms S's MRI demonstrated extensive white matter disease, although with relatively constant total brain volume. She was started on donepezil 5 mg at bedtime. Her dose was increased to 10 mg at bedtime 4 weeks later.

At her next follow-up visit, her mood remained euthymic. Her daughters noted an improved awareness of what was going on around her. Her MMSE score was 23, with errors in orientation and in following a 3-step command. Extended-release venlafaxine and donepezil were continued.

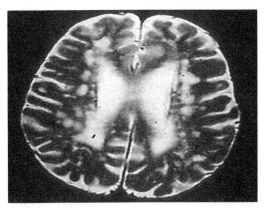

Fig. 1. MRI brain scan of a 73-year-old woman with major depression. The scan shows extensive white matter disease.

Depression, including MDD, remains a serious public health concern across the lifespan and especially in the elderly. Despite a lower overall percentage of depressed elders, when compared with their younger counterparts,[3] the expected increasing numbers of seniors point to an even greater necessity for health professionals to be aware of the specialized needs of elders.

The consequences of untreated or partially treated late-life depression are dire. There are higher mortality rates from both suicide[4] and medical illness.[5,6] Geriatric depression is also costly. In one study, total health care costs were 47% to 51% higher and outpatient costs were 43% to 52% higher for depressed elders when compared with non-depressed patients, even after adjustment for chronic medical illness. This increase was seen in every component of health care costs, with only a small percentage caused by mental health treatment.[7]

This issue of the *Psychiatric Clinics of North America* offers a comprehensive review of late-life depression. This article appraises several facets of geriatric depression, including a description of geriatric depression and recent epidemiologic studies highlighting the incidence and prevalence of old-age depression. The evidence regarding the cause of late-life depression is addressed from a biopsychosocial perspective. This review is crafted to be extensive, although not exhaustive. Particular attention is focused on vascular depression and the relationship between depression and cognitive impairment.

DESCRIPTION OF DEPRESSION IN OLDER ADULTS

Depression in older adults can have a variety of presentations: as recurrent disease stemming from earlier life (ie, early onset depression [EOD]); as new-onset depression (ie, late-onset depression [LOD]); as a mood disorder secondary to a general medical condition; or as mood symptoms secondary to substance or medication use. LOD is generally characterized as depression initially occurring past the age of 60–65.

Clinicians and clinical investigators do not agree as to what constitutes clinically significant depression nor is there universal agreement about how depression should be further divided into subtypes. The *Diagnostic and Statistical Manual of Mental Disorders* (Fourth Edition, Text Revision) (*DSM-IV-TR*) has set forth the criteria for assigning a diagnosis of MDD.[8] These criteria may change with the publication of the *Diagnostic and Statistical Manual of Mental Disorders* (Fifth Edition) in May of 2013.

Depressive states that do not meet the criteria for MDD can still result in significant impairment to the individual and in debilitating psychosocial effects. Several clinical depressive geriatric disorders have been described in the literature (**Table 1**).[8–11]

Minor depression or subthreshold depression is diagnosed when one of the core symptoms of depression is present along with 1 to 3 additional symptoms.[8] Minor depression and subthreshold depression in elders are of particular clinical importance because they have been associated with impairment similar to that of major depression, including impaired physical function, increased disability days, poorer self-rated health, perceived low social support, and excess service utilization.[10,12,13]

The depression–executive dysfunction syndrome has been thought of as major depression with prominent frontostriatal dysfunction. The syndrome is based on clinical, neuropathologic, and neuroimaging findings suggesting that frontostriatal dysfunction contributes to the development of both depression and executive dysfunction and influences the course of depression. Reduced verbal fluency, impaired visual naming, paranoia, loss of interest in activities, and psychomotor retardation characterize the syndrome. There is usually a rather mild associated vegetative pattern. Depressive signs and symptoms, especially psychomotor retardation and loss of interest in activities, contribute to disability in these patients. Depression with executive dysfunction has also been found to be associated with disability, poor treatment response, relapse, and recurrence.[11]

EPIDEMIOLOGY

The point prevalence estimates for MDD in elders in the community have been reported to be 4.4% in women and 2.7% in men in the Cache County Study.[14] The prevalence of either a major depressive episode or dysthymia in the Epidemiologic Catchment Area (ECA) survey was 2.5% in the geriatric age range.[3] A recent meta-analysis of older adults (aged 50 years and older) found a rate of 3.29% for current and 16.52% for lifetime MDD. For depressive symptoms, the prevalence rate was higher than for MDD, at 19.47%.[15] In 2012, the Institute of Medicine (IOM) published a report regarding the workforce for older adults (aged 65 years and older) with mental illness and/or substance use. The report made use of information from published research conducted in population-based samples in the United States as well as unpublished data. The committee found that the conditions with the highest prevalence among geriatric patients were depressive disorders, including a major depressive episode and dysthymic disorder. In 2010, about 1.2 million to 1.8 million

Table 1 Classification of geriatric depressive disorders	
MDD[8]	Mixed anxiety-depressive disorder[8]
Dysthymic disorder[8]	Bereavement[8]
Minor depressive disorder[8]	Adjustment disorder with depressed mood[8]
Depression without sadness[9]	Mood disorder caused by a general medical condition[8]
Subsyndromal or subthreshold depression[10]	(Vascular) dementia with depressed mood[8]
Depression–executive dysfunction syndrome[11]	Substance- or medication-induced depression[8]
Bipolar disorder, most recent episode depressed[8]	—

community-living older adults had these conditions. The 12-month prevalence rates were as follows: depressive disorders (3.0%–4.5%), major depressive episodes (3.0%–4.3%), dysthymic disorder (0.6%–1.6%), and depressive symptoms (1.1%–11.1%).[16]

Depression seems to both persist into older age as well as increase in prevalence through the geriatric age range. With respect to the oldest old (ie, elders aged 75 and greater) in a systematic review and meta-analysis, the pooled point prevalence of major depression was 7.2%. The rates of depression for women were between 4.0% and 10.3% and for men between 2.8% and 6.9% in the individual studies. The pooled prevalence of clinically significant depressive symptoms was 17.1%. The prevalence of clinically significant depressive symptoms increased in the higher age groups, by almost 20% to 25% in individuals aged 85 years and older and by about 30% to 50% in individuals aged 90 years and older, compared with those between 75 and 79 years of age, although no similar trend was found for major or minor depression.[17,18]

In the past several decades, many studies have examined the prevalence of late-life depression; however, there have been comparatively few incidence or new case studies. Lately, the first systematic review to examine this subject was completed. Twenty studies involving people aged 70 years and greater were reviewed. The incidence rate of MDD was found to be 0.2 to 14.1 per 100 person-years, and the incidence of clinically relevant depressive symptoms was 6.8 per 100 person-years. Female incidence was mostly higher than male incidence.[19]

The recurrence rates of depression were calculated in a new study. More than 5650 individuals were tracked in Rotterdam, Netherlands for 8 years on average. Recurrence for depressive symptoms and syndromes combined was 65.6 per 1000 patient-years. Recurrence was higher for women (73.1 per 1000 patient-years) than men (51.6 per 1000 patient-years). Recurrent episodes of depressive syndromes were almost equal between the genders, with an overall rate of 27.5 per 1000 patient-years.[20]

In the hospital and long-term-care settings, the frequency of major depression is much higher than in community settings. A total of 11.5% of hospitalized elders meet the criteria for MDD and 23% have depressive symptoms.[21] Major depression affects 5% to 10% of older adults in primary care settings.[22] The rates of major depression among nursing home residents are even higher. In one study of a long-term-care facility,[23] the prevalence estimate for probable and/or definite MDD was 14.4%. The estimate for minor depression was 16.8%. The prevalence of significant depressive signs and symptoms was 44.2%. Unfortunately, depression recognition was low; less than half of the cases diagnosed by psychiatrists were recognized as depressed by staff.[23] The IOM's report found an even higher prevalence of depression, 49.6%, among nursing home residents aged 65 years and older.[16]

MORTALITY

The consequences of elder depression are grim. There is both increased suicide and nonsuicide mortality. Although suicidal ideation decreases with age,[24] elders with suicidal thoughts are more likely to act on them and successfully commit suicide than their younger counterparts.[25] Older age has been significantly associated with more determined and planned self-destructive acts and with fewer warnings of suicidal intent.[24] Among those who attempt suicide, elders are the most likely to die. In adolescence, the ratio of attempted to completed suicides has been estimated to be 200:1, whereas the estimated risk for the general population is from 8:1 to 33:1. In contrast, there are approximately 4 attempts for each completed suicide in later life.[26] The most common mechanisms for suicide in a Canadian study involved firearms, hanging, self-poisoning, and falls from height,[27] which suggests increased lethality of self-destructive behaviors in older adults.[26]

Elder suicide remains a major public health crisis, and suicide has been overrepresented in this population. In 2004, the aged composed 12% of the US population, but elders accounted for 16% of suicide deaths. In 2010, 16.00 of every 100 000 people aged 65 years and older died by suicide, which was higher than the rate of 11.26 per 100 000 in the general population.[25] Suicide rates are highest among white men, rising in this population to a rate of more than 45 suicides per 100 000 per year. This number is 4 times the nation's overall age-adjusted rate.[28]

In addition to suicide, nonsuicide mortality is also a significant adverse outcome resulting from late-life depression. For adults aged 55 years and older in the New Haven ECA project,[29] the odds of dying were more than 4 times greater for individuals with affective disorders than for others, controlling for age, sex, and physical health. In a 7-year longitudinal follow-up of patients referred for geriatric psychiatry consultation, 50% of patients with Geriatric Depression Scale (GDS) scores greater than 6 died by 19 months versus 54 months for patients with GDS scores less than 7.[6] In a systematic review of the literature from 1997 to 2001, 72% of included studies demonstrated a positive association for depression with nonsuicide mortality, although a substantial minority did not. Depression may increase the likelihood of dying through several factors. Depressed people may be less likely to adhere to their medication regimen and maintain their cognitive and physical functioning capabilities, may be more likely to alienate their social network, and be less likely to seek out preventive and curative health care treatments.[30] In addition, depression itself may be harmful to the body. One of the most robust findings in the literature is the association of depression with increased mortality in those with cardiovascular disease.[6]

CONTRIBUTORS TO ELDER DEPRESSION

Many factors contribute to late-life depression, including biologic (**Table 2**) and psychosocial (**Table 3**). The biopsychosocial model[31] of understanding and organizing the cause of psychiatric illness has been useful in allowing mental health practitioners

Table 2
Biologic risk factors for late-life depression

Vascular	General health
Myocardial infarction	Obesity
Coronary heart disease	New medical illness
Hyperhomocysteinemia	Poor health status
Cerebrovascular accident	Poor self-perceived health
Silent cerebral infarction and white matter hyperintensities	
Genetic polymorphisms/mutations	Dementia
CADASIL	Alzheimer disease
MTHFR	Vascular dementia
CBS	
Diabetes mellitus	Parkinson disease

Abbreviations: CADASIL, cerebral autosomal dominant arteriopathy with subcortical infarcts and leukoencephalopathy; CBS, cystathionine beta-synthetase; MTHFR, methyltetrahydrofolate reductase.

Table 3 Psychosocial risk factors for late-life depression	
Personality attributes	Life stressors
Personality disorder	Stressful life events and daily hassles
Neuroticism	Medical illness and disability
Low level of self-efficacy	Poor functional status
Obsessional traits	Trauma
	Lower income
	Less education
Maladaptive thoughts and behaviors	Social stressors
Cognitive distortions	Perceived social support
Faulty information processing	Impaired social support
	Loneliness
Learned helplessness	Bereavement

to more easily and thoroughly conceptualize mental illness, although it may be unintentionally misleading in its separations. Elder depression, like depression in all age groups, likely stems from a complex multidirectional interaction of biologic, psychological (including personality based), and social factors.

Biologic Factors

Vascular depression

The vascular depression hypothesis is not new. Alexopoulos and colleagues[32] observed a characteristic cognitive pattern in depressed patients with vascular disease. In 1997, he coined the term *vascular depression* to describe these cases. The known comorbidity of depression, vascular disease, vascular risk factors, and the association of ischemic lesions with distinctive behavioral symptoms support the vascular depression hypothesis. Disruption of prefrontal systems or their modulating pathways by single lesions or by an accumulation of lesions exceeding a threshold are hypothesized to be the central mechanisms in vascular depression.[32] Symptomatically, these patients have more psychomotor retardation and less psychomotor agitation, less guilt, poorer insight, and limited depressive symptoms compared with controls. Cognitively, patients with vascular depression have greater overall cognitive impairment and disability than those with nonvascular depression. Fluency and naming are more impaired in patients with vascular depression.[33]

Several lines of evidence have led to the conclusion that cerebrovascular injury is linked to late-life depression. One line is the *homocysteine depression hypothesis*. Essentially, the hypothesis is that elevated levels of homocysteine lead to cerebral vascular disease and neurotransmitter deficiency, which then cause depressed mood. This linkage has been demonstrated in population and imaging studies. Levels of homocysteine may increase because of a multitude of factors, including dietary deficiency of B_{12}, folate, and B_6 and the genetic variation of enzymes, such as methyltetrahydrofolate reductase and cystathionine beta-synthetase, which are both essential for the metabolism of homocysteine.[34] The genetically based neurologic condition known as *cerebral autosomal dominant arteriopathy with subcortical infarcts and leukoencephalopathy* (CADASIL) many times arises with depression as one of its initial symptoms. The initial presentation, however, is primarily from either a stroke or a migraine; but up to 6% of patients may initially present with depression. Overall, psychiatric symptoms, including depression, adjustment disorder, and subcortical dementia, are present in up to 30% of patients with this ailment. The condition is caused by a mutation of the notch 3 gene.[35] Finally, several studies indicate that a large proportion of elderly persons with depression have had either a stroke or other evidence of cerebral compromise.[33,36] Many studies have also found high rates of cerebrovascular disease and white matter hyperintensities (WMH) on MRIs in depressed elderly patients.[37]

Neuroimaging has further added to the understanding of late-life depression. As a result, several areas of the brain have been implicated in late-life depression. These areas include the anterior cingulate cortex (ACC), orbitofrontal cortex (OFC), and the hippocampus.[38] In a meta-analysis of structures involved in depression, the ACC had the largest effect size. Depressed individuals had smaller ACC volumes.[39] The OFC functions as part of a network, which includes the hippocampus, amygdala, and basal ganglia. In elderly samples compared with nondepressed subjects, depressed patients have had smaller OFC volumes.[40] The hippocampus has been long associated with depression. As in the other implicated brain regions, studies in late-life depression have also demonstrated a reduction in hippocampal volume in the depressed elderly population.[39,41] Age of onset correlates negatively with hippocampal volume; patients with LOD have smaller volumes compared with those who have EOD and with controls.[41,42]

Functional neuroimaging has aided in the understanding of late-life depression. Regional cerebral blood flow and cerebral metabolism studies have demonstrated that the dorsal cingulate gyrus, middle and dorsolateral prefrontal cortex (DLPFC), insula, and superior temporal gyrus are all hypoactive at rest during negative mood states and that their activity increases with selective serotonin reuptake inhibitor treatment.[43] An additional network identified is a cortical-limbic network, which includes the medial and inferior frontal cortex and basal ganglia. These structures are overactive at rest and during induction of negative mood states. Their activity reduces with antidepressant treatment.[44] Overall, functional neuroimaging studies in late-life depression reveal a pattern of abnormal activation of frontolimbic regions, generally characterized by hypoactivation of specific dorsal cortical regions, including the DLPFC and the dorsal ACC, and hyperactivation of some limbic structures, such as the amygdala.[44] However, the bulk of the existent data are from midlife or mixed-age depression studies; it is possible that as more data become available, a different pattern may emerge in late life.[44]

It is thought that WMH are caused by small, silent cerebral infarctions. They are characterized by arteriosclerosis, perivascular demyelination, dilated periventricular spaces, and ischemia.[45,46] WMHs can predispose individuals to depression[32,37] by disrupting the fiber tracts connecting cortical and subcortical structures,[32] including tracts in the dorsolateral prefrontal cortex and the anterior cingulate cortex.[45] They are frequently found in patients with late-life depression.[37] In one study, among patients with late-life major depression, silent cerebral infarction was observed in 65.9% of those with EOD and in 93.7% of those with LOD.[47] A recent systematic review[48] confirmed this finding. The investigators found that WMHs are more common and severe in individuals with geriatric depression than in healthy controls and specifically in individuals with LOD. The odds of having white matter changes were more than 4 for LOD compared with EOD. Similarly, the severity of WMHs was greater in patients with LOD than in patients with EOD. The results supported the notion that LOD may be etiologically different from EOD.[48]

How might WMHs arise? Aside from known cerebrovascular risk factors,[49] new research has looked at the interrelationship of orthostatic blood pressure and WMH. In one study, participants with depression had a significantly larger decrease in systolic blood pressure on standing from a supine position than controls. The results indicated that depression might be an independent predictor for developing systolic orthostatic hypotension. Depressed participants also had lower-frequency heart rate variability and lower baroreflex sensitivity. Because brain MRI WMH are mostly ischemic, they may be associated with orthostatic blood pressure decreases.[50] In another study, an association between the degree of orthostatic systolic blood pressure decrease and WMH volume in depression was found.[51] The presence of autonomic abnormalities in late-life depression could partly be associated with the development of and/or worsening of WMH and late-life depression.

Relationship of late-life depression and cognitive impairment
It has long been known that a relationship exists between memory impairment and depression,[52] although the nature of this relationship has been unclear.[53] Although in the past cognitive impairment related to depression has been thought to reverse with remission of depression, it now seems that there may be longer-lasting effects. In one study, over 3 years, irreversible dementia developed significantly more frequently in the depressed group with the dementia syndrome of depression (DSD) (43%) than in the group with depression alone (12%). The group with DSD had a 4.69-times higher chance of having developed dementia at follow-up than the patients with depression alone.[54] A meta-analysis, which compared patients with depression with those with Alzheimer dementia, found neuropsychological deficiencies on almost every psychological test among patients with depression. Many of the deficits, such as with recall or on recognition tasks, were no different than those seen in patients suffering from dementia. These findings are not consistent with the hypothesis that depression is merely associated with deficits in effortful processing but rather suggest a more pervasive and insidious process at play in depressed elders.[55] Research of this nature has led to a series of questions concerning the nature of the relationship between depression and memory impairment. A few questions include the following: Is depression a symptom of dementia? Does a history of depression constitute a risk factor for later dementia? Can depression be a prodrome of dementia?[2] What is the relationship between vascular depression and vascular dementia?

Symptoms or syndromes of depression are often present in dementia and may constitute one of the many behavioral and psychological symptoms of dementia.[2] A sizable minority of patients with Alzheimer disease, during the course of their disorder, will exhibit depressed mood (40%–50%) whereas actual depressive disorders are encountered in about 10% to 20%.[56] Depression may occur more commonly as a symptom in vascular dementia than in Alzheimer dementia.[57]

Risk factor for dementia Data regarding depression as a risk factor for dementia have been mixed[53,58]; however, some tentative conclusions can be drawn from the available evidence. In a recent meta-analysis of 12 longitudinal studies, patients with depression had higher rates of Alzheimer dementia (AD), vascular dementia (VD), any dementia, and mild cognitive impairment (MCI) than those without depression. The relative risk for the associations ranged from 1.55 for any dementia to 1.97 for MCI.[59] Another recent large systematic review and meta-analysis confirmed this finding and found that a history of depression increased the odds of later developing AD by 2.02.[60] The interval between diagnoses of depression and AD was positively related to increased risk of developing AD, suggesting that rather than a prodrome, depression may be a risk factor for AD.[60] This risk also extends into later age, and depression remains a risk factor for cognitive impairment even among the oldest old.[61] Recurrent depression seems to present a greater risk for dementia than a single depressive episode, such that patients with many prior hospitalizations for depression have an increased risk of developing subsequent dementia. On average, each depressive episode is associated with a 13% increased rate of dementia.[62] Taken together, these findings suggest that depression is indeed a risk factor for dementia and that earlier-onset, recurrent disease confers the greatest risk for the subsequent development of cognitive impairment.

Cause of dementia Beyond serving as a risk factor for dementia, depression could play a causative role in the development of dementia. A possible mechanism is suggested by the glucocorticoid hypothesis.[63] According to this idea, a prolonged physical reaction to stress, such as that associated with a major depressive episode, elicits sustained glucocorticoid secretion. There are glucocorticoid receptors in the hippocampus. Over time, glucocorticoid hypersecretion leads to excessive activation of hippocampal glucocorticoid receptors, which is toxic to the hippocampus and leads to hippocampal atrophy. Such damage has been recorded in imaging studies[41] and has been associated with dementia.[64]

The hypothesis that depression is a prodrome to dementia is most compatible with studies, of which there are many, in which depression occurs close in time to the onset of dementia.[53,65,66] It is conceivable that many cases of late-life depression could be an early prodromal sign of dementia, especially because the pathologic changes of dementing diseases can begin long before their onset.[67] However, if depression were a prodrome to dementia, then its presence should reliably predict future cognitive disturbance.[2]

Vascular depression Lastly, turning to vascular depression and its relationship to vascular dementia, owing to the similarity of risk factors for the two conditions, a connection between them would seem reasonable; however, the path from vascular disease to vascular depression to vascular dementia is likely reciprocal and not direct or sequential.[68] Little research has been completed to elucidate this question. A case report suggests that such a relationship may exist.[69] The PAQUID study[66] documented that the risk for dementia was 50% higher in depressed men with hypertension compared with depressed nonhypertensive men. It seems from this study that in some men, vascular disease leads to depressive symptoms and that a subgroup of those who develop depression progress to dementia.[66] Barnes and colleagues[70] found that subjects with midlife and late life symptoms had more than a 3-fold increase in vascular dementia risk, whereas subjects with late-life depressive symptoms had a 2-fold increase in AD risk. Barnes and colleagues[70] also found that late-life depressive symptoms were more predictive of dementia than early life depressive symptoms, although other analyses, as mentioned, have yielded different results.[58]

Thus, given these findings, it seems likely that depression is a risk factor for dementia. Evidence to support this is plentiful,[59,60,70] but there are also opposing studies.[66] EOD may confer a greater risk of dementia than LOD,[58,65] although other studies have concluded the opposite.[70] The greatest risk for dementia probably exists in those with both midlife and late-life depression.[70] There is also a dose-response relationship between depression and dementia, such that each depressive episode is associated with an increased rate of dementia.[62] At the same time, some cases of LOD undoubtedly represent a prodromal symptom of dementia.[58] Ultimately, depression probably serves as both a risk factor and at times a prodromal symptom for dementia.

Medical comorbidity

Late-life depression often arises in the context of medical and neurologic illness.[71] According to the *DSM-IV-TR*, MDD cannot be diagnosed when symptoms are the direct physiologic result of a medical condition.[8] As a result, depression may be either underdiagnosed or overdiagnosed in the presence of conditions such as cancer that can also cause weight loss, fatigue, poor appetite, and/or disruption of sleep.

Although almost any serious or chronic condition can produce a depressive reaction, the disorders that are most strongly associated with depression include cardiac conditions and neurologic illness, including cerebrovascular disease. Specific medical conditions that may be associated with geriatric depression include myocardial infarction, coronary heart disease, cardiac catheterization,[72] diabetes,[73] obesity, and body mass index.[74] Approximately 20% to 25% of patients with heart disease experience major depression, and another 20% to 25% report symptoms of depression.[72] In the IOM's report, in community-living adults aged 60 years and older who had major depression or dysthymia, the most common coexisting physical health conditions were hypertension (58%), chronic pain (57%), arthritis (56%), loss of hearing or vision (55%), urinary tract and prostate disease (39%), heart disease (28%), and diabetes (23%).[16] Substances that have been linked to old-age depression include methyldopa, benzodiazepines, propranolol, reserpine, steroids, anti-Parkinsonian agents, β-blockers, cimetidine, clonidine, hydralazine, estrogens, progesterone, tamoxifen, vinblastine, vincristine, and dextropropoxyphene.[75] New medical illness, poor health status, and poor self-perceived health also increase the risk for depression.[76]

Neurologic disorders

High rates of cerebrovascular disease and other neurologic disorders have been associated with elder depression. In patients who have had a stroke, the prevalence rate for major depression is 19.3% among hospitalized patients and 23.3% in outpatients.[36] Silent cerebral infarctions are observed in many patients with EOD or LOD.[47]

The rate of depression among those with Parkinson disease (PD) is high. The prevalence of MDD in patients with PD varies from 7.7% in population studies to more than 25% in outpatient samples.[77] Depressive symptoms occur in approximately half of the patients with PD and are a significant cause of functional impairment. There is accumulating evidence suggesting that depression in PD is secondary to underlying neuroanatomical degeneration, which results in changes in central serotonergic function and in neurodegeneration of specific cortical and subcortical pathways rather than simply a reaction to psychosocial stress and disability.[78] Depression in PD may be a milder form of depression and is less frequently associated with dysphoria, anhedonia, feelings of guilt, and loss of energy but is associated with more concentration problems than depression in older adults without neurologic disease.[77] In order to avoid underdiagnosing depression in PD, a study group has proposed a specific syndrome, depression of PD, and has recommended an inclusive approach that considers all symptoms as related to depression, regardless of their overlap with PD or other medical conditions.[79]

Psychosocial Factors

Psychological and social variables are often intertwined. They may be just as important as physical factors in understanding the elements leading to late-life depression. For example, in institutionalized elders, psychological variables, such as environmental mastery (a sense of self-efficacy and competence in managing one's environment), purpose in life, and autonomy, had a greater importance in understanding depression than traditional risk factors, such as medical illness and disability. These 3 psychological variables discriminated between patients with and without MDD 80% of the time.[80] This section reviews the roles of personality attributes, behavior, cognition, psychodynamic theory, social support, and life stressors in elder depression.

Personality attributes

Neuroticism is an enduring tendency to experience negative emotional states. Those who score high on neuroticism scales are more likely to respond poorly to stress and to interpret situations as threatening or hopelessly difficult. Increasingly, it is being recognized as a significant public health concern.[81] Neuroticism has been associated with late-life depression. Of 1511 nondepressed elderly respondents (aged 55–85 years at baseline) in the Longitudinal Aging Study Amsterdam, 17% developed a clinically relevant level of depressive symptoms during a 6-year follow-up period. Personality, neuroticism in particular, was found to be a consistent and important predictor of the onset of depressive symptoms in late life. It was an even more important predictor of depression than health-related and situational factors, with a relative risk for prediction of 3.6. Aging did not affect the strength of the association. Other personality factors that played an important role in predicting depression were mastery and self-efficacy.[82] In a follow-up study, personality aberrations were also associated with recurrence of depression in later life. In particular, neuroticism and a low level of mastery were noted as contributing factors, along with residual depressive symptoms at the time of recovery, female gender, pain complaints, and feelings of loneliness.[83]

Other personality attributes that may contribute to late-life depression include the presence of a personality disorder, attachment style, and obsessional traits. The frequency of strictly diagnosable personality disorders shows only a small decline with aging.[84] Patients with a personality disorder are almost 4 times more likely to experience maintenance or reemergence of significant depressive symptoms than those without a personality disorder. In addition to a personality disorder, hopelessness and ambivalence regarding emotional expression also predict the maintenance or reemergence of depressive symptoms.[85] Insecure attachment is another risk factor for developing new depression. In elders and older adults, both patients with EOD and LOD showed greater insecure attachment and poorer social adaption compared with never-depressed controls. No difference was found between patients with EOD and LOD in attachment style or social adaptation.[86] Obsessional traits seem to affect suicide risk, possibly because they may undermine an elder's ability to cope with the challenges of aging, which often call for substantial adaptations.[87]

Behavior
Learned helplessness is the idea that the cause of depression is the expectation that initiating action in a continually stressful environment is futile.[88] A reformulation of the model attributes depression to the belief that highly desired outcomes are improbable or highly aversive outcomes are probable and that the individual expects that no response in their repertoire will change that likelihood. These beliefs about oneself and one's environment lead to helplessness and depression.[88]

Unfortunately, elders frequently face circumstances that can produce thought patterns that may lead to learned helplessness. As the result of aging, they may feel helpless against the onslaught of recurrent and uncontrollable physical illness and its effects on them and to changes in their social position. This notion has several supporting elements from the literature. For example, poor functional status secondary to physical illness is among the most important of the causes of depressive symptoms in older adults. Disability has been conceptualized as a chronic and stressful condition that may provoke reactions, such as feelings of worthlessness or hopelessness that ultimately contribute to depression.[89] Next, the total number of life events and the total number of daily hassles is strongly associated with depression, although sudden unexpected events have not been related to depression.[90] Again, the chronicity and perceived uncontrollability of these events could contribute to depression. Lastly, longitudinal cohort studies have identified several other significant psychosocial risk factors for late-life depressive disorders. Some of these have included long-standing situations, such as ongoing difficulties; medical illness and injuries; disability and functional decline; and lack of social contacts.[91]

Cognition

Cognitive behavior therapy is based on the idea that mental illness is the product of maladaptive thoughts and behaviors and that a 2-way relationship between cognition and behavior exists in which cognitive processes can influence behavior and behavioral change can influence cognitions.[92] Further, it posits that faulty information processing and unhelpful behaviors lead to mental illness, including depressed mood states.[93] A negative mood state is produced when information processing is highly negatively biased and frequently inaccurate[94] because of distorted patterns of thinking and/or errors in logic.[92] Aaron Beck and colleagues[93] noted a distinctive pattern of thinking in depressed patients that was characterized by a global negative view of themselves, the outside world, and the future. This cognitive triad is the following: I am defective. The world is a hostile place. Things will never change.[93] Negative thinking further influences behavior so that patients' social and interpersonal functioning deteriorates. These behavioral changes then help to confirm patients' negative viewpoints, thereby reinforcing themselves.[94]

There is evidence that elders with depression experience cognitive distortions. In one study, cognitive coping strategies seemed to play an important role in relation to depressive symptoms in late life. Elderly people with more depressive symptoms were reported to use rumination and catastrophizing to a significantly higher extent and positive reappraisal to a significantly lower extent than those with lower depression scores.[95] Enhanced sensitivity to negative feedback also occurs in mild late-life depression[96] and could stem from the belief that one is defective. Lastly, just as in learned helplessness, chronic stressors could serve to reinforce the outlook that the world is hostile and things will never change, ultimately leading to hopelessness, withdrawal, and depression.

Psychodynamic theory

A psychodynamic understanding of depression is not a unitary concept and can be approached from many different perspectives. One is that depression results from introjected (inwardly directed) anger regarding a lost relationship with an important person who has become unavailable, potentially through relocation or death. In depression, or melancholia, what feels lost or damaged is part of the self,[97] such that the ego itself is seen as poor and empty rather than the world, as is the case in mourning.[98]

In depressed elders, loss is not an uncommon experience because loss and coping with loss are regrettably part of the aging process. Under this facet of psychodynamic theory, elders who internalize their negative emotions may be more likely to become depressed. Although grief and bereavement in elders have not been linked specifically to psychodynamic theory, one example of this may be complicated bereavement.[16] Studies have found that bereavement is associated with depressive symptoms in older adults and may be one of the most significant risk factors for depression in late life.[99] In one study, the risk of depression associated with the death of one's spouse increased the adjusted odds of depression by 12.1 and of dysphoria by 21.8.[100] Another study looked at 1810 community-dwelling older adults who were aged 55 years and older. After 3 years, 9% of the subjects had scored beyond the thresholds for symptoms of depression and anxiety. Vulnerability for depression and anxiety was quite similar, but life events differed. The onset of depression was predicted by death of a partner or other relatives, whereas the onset of anxiety was best predicted by having a partner who developed a major illness.[101] These studies did not examine psychological interpretations of these events, but it seems clear that the loss of an important relationship had an important effect, for a myriad of reasons, on the subsequent development of depression.

Social support

Social relationships, ranging from social isolation to social support, have long been implicated in the risk for depression. Social support is a multifactorial construct. It involves dimensions of perception, structure, and behavior. Social isolation and impaired social support have been associated with moderate and severe depressive symptoms in the elderly.[102] The most vigorous findings involve perceived support, also called *emotional support*. Perceived social support has proved to be among the most robust predictors of late-life depressive symptoms.[91] A study from Hong Kong[103] found that a significant relationship existed between social support and depressive signs and symptoms on all dimensions of social support, including social network size, network composition, social contact frequency, satisfaction of social support, instrumental/emotional support, and helping others. However, again, satisfaction with support was a more important predictor of depression than the other objective measures of network relationships. The consequences of impaired social relationships can be significant because the absence of a friend or a confidante can contribute to suicidal behavior in elders.[104]

Elders may keenly feel the effects of loneliness. Loneliness has been defined by one group as the absence of a sense of integration into the social environment or as a lower level of perceived emotional togetherness in social interactions. Elders who are lonely are more depressed and experience less togetherness than those who are not lonely.[105] The risk of depression caused by a lack of contact with friends has been estimated to be 2.5, and the risk of depression caused by loneliness has been calculated to be 3.6.[106]

Life stressors

Longitudinal cohort studies have identified several stressors that serve as risk factors for late-life depressive disorders. These stressors include adverse life events and ongoing difficulties; death of a spouse or other loved one; medical illness, especially diseases of the cardiovascular system, and injuries; and disability and functional decline.[91,99] For community-dwelling older adults, the presence of disabilities, measured by an Activities of Daily Living Score of 1 to 4, increased the risk of depression by 3.7 over 1 year, after adjusting for age, gender, marital status, loneliness, contact with friends, and index depression score.[106] As noted previously, the loss of a loved one is one of the most significant risk factors for late-life depression. How one copes with the loss, how traumatic or unexpected the death is, and the degree to which the death results in social isolation might be some of the linking features between loss and new-onset depression.[99] Trauma and fear of victimization are relatively understudied potential sources of depression in elders. They may be related to the onset of late-life depression through the behavioral consequences of fear[99] and avoidance.

Aside from acute life events, chronic stressors can also influence the development of late-life depression. Some stressors include lower income[99] and less education,[107] as well as those previously mentioned. Lower income is related to poorer access to health and mental health services.[99] When compared with elders with more education, those with less education have a higher risk of depression, with a relative risk of 1.49.[107]

Life stressors can arouse negative emotional states in elders in many ways. They can be profoundly psychologically meaningful and may considerably disrupt one's life. They often necessitate change and readjustment. They can also precipitate hospitalization, reduce social activities, increase disability, shift the nature of social relationships, or even result in residential relocation.[91] Maladaptive coping strategies, including unhelpful patterns of thinking and behaving, for stressful events can lead to dysphoric mood states. Symptoms may be influenced by characteristic beliefs, including the viewpoint that highly aversive outcomes are probable and that no response will change their likelihood. An elder's ability to adapt to change could be swayed by negative beliefs about oneself and one's ability to control the environment or manage future events. The presence of a personality disorder, or neuroticism, can also impair one's ability to manage. Poor social support can decrease psychological resilience and foster a depressive response to life stressors. Impairment in any of these areas could lead to the persistence of depressive symptoms and/or syndromes.

SUMMARY

Depression in the elderly is a complex disorder. In many ways, it is the quintessential biopsychosocial disorder. There is a great deal of literature linking structural brain changes to late-life depression, but even recent meta-analyses note the heterogeneity of findings and call for further research.[108] Psychological factors in depression remain salient across the lifespan, but older adults face new social challenges. For clinicians seeking to manage aging depressed patients, the multiplicity of factors contributing to the presentation is challenging and demands a holistic perspective. Researchers must also account for biologic, psychological, and social factors as they seek to understand the underpinnings of depression in the elderly. The encouraging news for clinicians and researchers is that much work has been done that not only yields clinical insights but also provides a direction for future studies.

REFERENCES

1. Werner C. The older population: 2010. 2011. Available at: http://2010.census. gov/2010census/. Accessed November 21, 2012.
2. Ellison JM, Kyomen HH, Harper DG. Depression in later life: an overview with treatment recommendations. Psychiatr Clin North Am 2012;35(1):203–29.
3. Regier DA, Boyd JH, Burke JD Jr, et al. One-month prevalence of mental disorders in the United States based on five epidemiologic catchment area sites. Arch Gen Psychiatry 1988;45(11):977–86.
4. Mitty E, Flores S. Suicide in late life. Geriatr Nurs 2008;29(3):160–5.
5. Frasure-Smith N, Lesperance F, Talajic M. Depression following myocardial infarction: impact on 6-month survival. JAMA 1993;270(15):1819–25.
6. Royall DR, Schillerstrom JE, Piper PK, et al. Depression and mortality in elders referred for geriatric psychiatry consultation. J Am Med Dir Assoc 2007;8(5): 318–21.
7. Katon WJ, Lin E, Russo J, et al. Increased medical costs of a population-based sample of depressed elderly patients. Arch Gen Psychiatry 2003;60(9):897–903.
8. American Psychiatric Association. Diagnostic and statistical manual of mental disorders: DSM-IV-TR. Washington, DC: American Psychiatric Publishing, Inc; 2000.
9. Gallo JJ, Rabins PV, Lyketsos CG, et al. Depression without sadness: functional outcomes of nondysphoric depression in later life. J Am Geriatr Soc 1997;45(5): 570–8.

10. Lavretsky H, Kumar A. Clinically significant non-major depression. Am J Geriatr Psychiatry 2002;10(3):239–55.
11. Alexopoulos GS, Kiosses DN, Klimstra S, et al. Clinical presentation of the "depression-executive dysfunction syndrome" of late life. Am J Geriatr Psychiatry 2002;10(1):98–106.
12. Beekman AT, Deeg DJ, Braam AW, et al. Consequences of major and minor depression in later life- a study of disability, well-being, and service utilization. Psychol Med 1997;27(6):1397–409.
13. Hybels CF, Blazer DG, Pieper CF. Toward a threshold for subthreshold depression: an analysis of correlates of depression by severity of symptoms using data from an elderly community sample. Gerontologist 2001;41(3):357–65.
14. Steffens DC, Skoog I, Norton MC, et al. Prevalence of depression and its treatment in an elderly population: the cache county study. Arch Gen Psychiatry 2000;57(6):601–7.
15. Volkert J, Schulz H, Harter M, et al. The prevalence of mental disorders in older people in Western countries-a meta-analysis. Ageing Res Rev 2012;12(1):339–53.
16. IOM (Institute of Medicine). The mental health and substance use workforce for older adults: in whose hands? Washington, DC: The National Academies Press; 2012.
17. Leach LS. Review: major depression affects about 7% of adults aged 75 and above. Evid Based Ment Health 2012;15(3):64.
18. Luppa M, Sikorski C, Luck T, et al. Age- and gender-specific prevalence of depression in latest-life–systematic review and meta-analysis. J Affect Disord 2012;136(3):212–21.
19. Büchtemann D, Luppa M, Bramesfeld A, et al. Incidence of late-life depression: a systematic review. J Affect Disord 2012;142(1–3):172–9.
20. Luijendijk HJ, van den Berg JF, Dekker MJ, et al. Incidence and recurrence of late-life depression. Arch Gen Psychiatry 2008;65(12):1394–401.
21. Koenig HG, Meador KG, Cohen HJ, et al. Depression in elderly hospitalized patients with medical illness. Arch Intern Med 1988;148(9):1929–36.
22. Blazer DG. Depression in late life: review and commentary. J Gerontol A Biol Sci Med Sci 2003;58(3):M249–65.
23. Teresi J, Abrams R, Holmes D, et al. Prevalence of depression and depression recognition in nursing homes. Soc Psychiatry Psychiatr Epidemiol 2001;36(12):613–20.
24. Conwell Y, Duberstein PR, Cox C, et al. Age differences in behaviors leading to completed suicide. Am J Geriatr Psychiatry 1998;6(2):122–6.
25. Centers for Disease Control and Prevention (CDC), editor. Web-based injury statistics query and reporting system (WISQARS) [Online]. 2010. Available at: http://www.cdc.gov/injury/wisqars/index.html. Accessed November 23, 2012.
26. Conwell Y, Duberstein PR, Caine ED. Risk factors for suicide in later life. Biol Psychiatry 2002;52(3):193–204.
27. Juurlink DN, Herrmann N, Szalai JP, et al. Medical illness and the risk of suicide in the elderly. Arch Intern Med 2004;164(11):1179.
28. Conwell Y, Van Orden K, Caine ED. Suicide in older adults. Psychiatr Clin North Am 2011;34(2):451–68.
29. Bruce ML, Leaf PJ. Psychiatric disorders and 15-month mortality in a community sample of older adults. Am J Public Health 1989;79(6):727–30.
30. Schulz R, Drayer RA, Rollman BL. Depression as a risk factor for non-suicide mortality in the elderly. Biol Psychiatry 2002;52(3):205–25.

31. Engel G. The clinical application of the biopsychosocial model. Am J Psychiatry 1980;137:535–44.
32. Alexopoulos GS, Meyers BS, Young RC, et al. 'Vascular depression' hypothesis. Arch Gen Psychiatry 1997;54(10):915–22.
33. Alexopoulos GS, Meyers BS, Young RC, et al. Clinically defined vascular depression. Am J Psychiatry 1997;154(4):562–5.
34. Folstein M, Liu T, Peter I, et al. The homocysteine hypothesis of depression. Am J Psychiatry 2007;164(6):861–7.
35. Taylor MA, Doody GA. CADASIL: a guide to a comparatively unrecognised condition in psychiatry. Adv Psychiatr Treat 2008;14(5):350–7.
36. Robinson RG. Poststroke depression: prevalence, diagnosis, treatment, and disease progression. Biol Psychiatry 2003;54(3):376–87.
37. Culang-Reinlieb ME, Johnert LC, Brickman AM, et al. MRI-defined vascular depression: a review of the construct. Int J Geriatr Psychiatry 2011;26(11):1101–8.
38. Benjamin S, Steffens DC. Structural neuroimaging of geriatric depression. Psychiatr Clin North Am 2011;34(2):423–35, ix.
39. Koolschijn PC, van Haren NE, Lensvelt-Mulders GJ, et al. Brain volume abnormalities in major depressive disorder: a meta-analysis of magnetic resonance imaging studies. Hum Brain Mapp 2009;30(11):3719–35.
40. Taylor WD, Macfall JR, Payne ME, et al. Orbitofrontal cortex volume in late life depression: influence of hyperintense lesions and genetic polymorphisms. Psychol Med 2007;37(12):1763–73.
41. Steffens DC, Byrum CE, McQuoid DR, et al. Hippocampal volume in geriatric depression. Biol Psychiatry 2000;48(4):301–9.
42. Lloyd AJ, Ferrier IN, Barber R, et al. Hippocampal volume change in depression: late- and early-onset illness compared. Br J Psychiatry 2004;184:488–95.
43. Fitzgerald PB, Laird AR, Maller J, et al. A meta-analytic study of changes in brain activation in depression. Hum Brain Mapp 2008;29(6):683–95.
44. Gunning FM, Smith GS. Functional neuroimaging in geriatric depression. Psychiatr Clin North Am 2011;34(2):403–22, viii.
45. Thomas AJ, O'Brien JT, Davis S, et al. Ischemic basis for deep white matter hyperintensities in major depression: a neuropathological study. Arch Gen Psychiatry 2002;59(9):785.
46. Fazekas F, Kleinert R, Offenbacher H, et al. Pathologic correlates of incidental MRI white matter signal hyperintensities. Neurology 1993;43(9):1683–9.
47. Fujikawa T, Yamawaki S, Touhouda Y. Incidence of silent cerebral infarction in patients with major depression. Stroke 1993;24(11):1631–4.
48. Herrmann LL, Le Masurier M, Ebmeier KP. White matter hyperintensities in late life depression: a systematic review. J Neurol Neurosurg Psychiatry 2008;79(6):619–24.
49. Greenwald BS, Kramer-Ginsberg E, Krishnan RR, et al. MRI signal hyperintensities in geriatric depression. Am J Psychiatry 1996;153(9):1212.
50. Vasudev A, O'Brien JT, Tan MP, et al. A study of orthostatic hypotension, heart rate variability and baroreflex sensitivity in late-life depression. J Affect Disord 2011;131(1–3):374–8.
51. Colloby SJ, Vasudev A, O'Brien JT, et al. Relationship of orthostatic blood pressure to white matter hyperintensities and subcortical volumes in late-life depression. Br J Psychiatry 2011;199(5):404–10.
52. Burt DB, Zembar MJ, Niederehe G. Depression and memory impairment: a meta-analysis of the association, its pattern, and specificity. Psychol Bull 1995;117(2):285.

53. Jorm AF. History of depression as a risk factor for dementia: an updated review. Aust N Z J Psychiatry 2001;35(6):776–81.
54. Alexopoulos GS, Meyers BS, Young RC, et al. The course of geriatric depression with "reversible dementia": a controlled study. Am J Psychiatry 1993;150:1693–9.
55. Christensen H, Griffiths K, MacKinnon A, et al. A quantitative review of cognitive deficits in depression and Alzheimer-type dementia. J Int Neuropsychol Soc 1997;3(06):631–51.
56. Wragg RE, Jeste DV. Overview of depression and psychosis in Alzheimer's disease. Am J Psychiatry 1989;146(5):577–87.
57. Newman SC. The prevalence of depression in Alzheimer's disease and vascular dementia in a population sample. J Affect Disord 1999;52(1):169–76.
58. Kessing LV. Depression and the risk for dementia. Curr Opin Psychiatry 2012; 25(6):457–61.
59. Gao Y, Huang C, Zhao K, et al. Depression as a risk factor for dementia and mild cognitive impairment: a meta-analysis of longitudinal studies. Int J Geriatr Psychiatry 2013;28(5):441–9.
60. Ownby RL, Crocco E, Acevedo A, et al. Depression and risk for Alzheimer disease: systematic review, meta-analysis, and metaregression analysis. Arch Gen Psychiatry 2006;63(5):530.
61. Spira AP, Rebok GW, Stone KL, et al. Depressive symptoms in oldest-old women: risk of mild cognitive impairment and dementia. Am J Geriatr Psychiatry 2012;20(12):1006–15.
62. Kessing LV, Andersen PK. Does the risk of developing dementia increase with the number of episodes in patients with depressive disorder and in patients with bipolar disorder? J Neurol Neurosurg Psychiatry 2004;75(12):1662–6.
63. Sapolsky RM, Krey LC, McEwen BS. The neuroendocrinology of stress and aging: the glucocorticoid cascade hypothesis. Sci Aging Knowledge Environ 2002;2002(38):21.
64. Seab JP, Jagust WJ, Wong ST, et al. Quantitative NMR measurements of hippocampal atrophy in Alzheimer's disease. Magn Reson Med 2005;8(2):200–8.
65. Jorm AF, Van Duijn CM, Chandra V, et al. Psychiatric history and related exposures as risk factors for Alzheimer's disease: a collaborative re-analysis of case-control studies. Int J Epidemiol 1991;20(Suppl 2):S43–7.
66. Fuhrer R, Dufouil C, Dartigues JF. Exploring sex differences in the relationship between depressive symptoms and dementia incidence: prospective results from the PAQUID Study. J Am Geriatr Soc 2003;51(8):1055–63.
67. Bateman RJ, Xiong C, Benzinger TL, et al. Clinical and biomarker changes in dominantly inherited Alzheimer's disease. N Engl J Med 2012;367(9):795–804.
68. Alexopoulos GS. Vascular disease, depression, and dementia. J Am Geriatr Soc 2003;51(8):1178–80.
69. Steffens DC, Taylor WD, Krishnan KR. Progression of subcortical ischemic disease from vascular depression to vascular dementia. Am J Psychiatry 2003; 160(10):1751–6.
70. Barnes DE, Yaffe K, Byers AL, et al. Midlife vs late-life depressive symptoms and risk of dementia: differential effects for Alzheimer disease and vascular dementia. Arch Gen Psychiatry 2012;69(5):493–8.
71. Alexopoulos GS, Buckwalter K, Olin J, et al. Comorbidity of late life depression: an opportunity for research on mechanisms and treatment. Biol Psychiatry 2002; 52(6):543–58.
72. Carney RM, Freedland KE. Depression, mortality, and medical morbidity in patients with coronary heart disease. Biol Psychiatry 2003;54(3):241–7.

73. Blazer DG, Moody-Ayers S, Craft-Morgan J, et al. Depression in diabetes and obesity- racial: ethnic: gender issues in older adults. J Psychosom Res 2002; 53(4):913–6.
74. Sachs-Ericsson N, Burns AB, Gordon KH, et al. Body mass index and depressive symptoms in older adults- the moderating roles of race, sex, and socioeconomic status. Am J Geriatr Psychiatry 2007;15(9):815–25.
75. Alexopoulos GS. Depression in the elderly. Lancet 2005;365(9475):1961–70.
76. Cole MG, Dendukuri N. Risk factors for depression among elderly community subjects: a systematic review and meta-analysis. Am J Psychiatry 2003;160(6): 1147–56.
77. Ehrt U, Brønnick K, Leentjens AF, et al. Depressive symptom profile in Parkinson's disease: a comparison with depression in elderly patients without Parkinson's disease. Int J Geriatr Psychiatry 2006;21(3):252–8.
78. McDonald WM, Richard IH, DeLong MR. Prevalence, etiology, and treatment of depression in Parkinson's disease. Biol Psychiatry 2003;54(3):363.
79. Marsh L, McDonald WM, Cummings J, et al. Provisional diagnostic criteria for depression in Parkinson's disease: report of an NINDS/NIMH Work Group. Mov Disord 2005;21(2):148–58.
80. Davison TE, McCabe MP, Knight T, et al. Biopsychosocial factors related to depression in aged care residents. J Affect Disord 2012;142(1–3):290–6.
81. Lahey BB. Public health significance of neuroticism. Am Psychol 2009;64(4):241.
82. Steunenberg B, Beekman AT, Deeg DJ, et al. Personality and the onset of depression in late life. J Affect Disord 2006;92(2–3):243–51.
83. Steunenberg B, Beekman AT, Deeg DJ, et al. Personality predicts recurrence of late-life depression. J Affect Disord 2010;123(1–3):164–72.
84. Abrams RC, Bromberg CE. Personality disorders in the elderly: a flagging field of inquiry. Int J Geriatr Psychiatry 2006;21(11):1013–7.
85. Morse JQ, Lynch TR. A preliminary investigation of self-reported personality disorders in late life: prevalence, predictors of depressive severity, and clinical correlates. Aging Ment Health 2004;8(4):307–15.
86. Paradiso S, Naridze R, Holm-Brown E. Lifetime romantic attachment style and social adaptation in late-onset depression. Int J Geriatr Psychiatry 2012; 27(10):1008–16.
87. Hawton K, van Heeringen K. Suicide. Lancet 2009;373(9672):1372–81.
88. Abramson LY, Seligman ME, Teasdale JD. Learned helplessness in humans: critique and reformulation. J Abnorm Psychol 1978;87(1):49.
89. Bruce ML. Depression and disability in late life: directions for future research. Am J Geriatr Psychiatry 2001;9(2):102–12.
90. Kraaij V, Arensman E, Spinhoven P. Negative life events and depression in elderly persons a meta-analysis. J Gerontol B Psychol Sci Soc Sci 2002;57(1): P87–94.
91. Bruce ML. Psychosocial risk factors for depressive disorders in late life. Biol Psychiatry 2002;52(3):175–84.
92. Wright JH. Cognitive behavior therapy: basic principles and recent advances. Focus 2006;4(2):173.
93. Beck AT, Rush AJ, Shaw BF, et al. Cognitive therapy of depression. United States of America: The Guilford Press; 1987.
94. Sudak DM. Cognitive behavioral therapy for depression. Psychiatr Clin North Am 2012;35(1):99–110.
95. Kraaij V, Pruymboom E, Garnefski N. Cognitive coping and depressive symptoms in the elderly: a longitudinal study. Aging Ment Health 2002;6(3):275–81.

96. von Gunten A, Herrmann FR, Elliott R, et al. Abnormal sensitivity to negative feedback in late-life depression. Psychiatry Clin Neurosci 2011;65(4):333–40.

97. McWilliams N. Psychoanalytic diagnosis: understanding personality structure in the clinical process. United States of America: Guilford Press; 2011.

98. Freud S. Mourning and melancholia. London: The Hogarth Press; 1917.

99. Areán PA, Reynolds CF III. The impact of psychosocial factors on late-life depression. Biol Psychiatry 2005;58(4):277–82.

100. Bruce ML, Kim K, Leaf PJ, et al. Depressive episodes and dysphoria resulting from conjugal bereavement in a prospective community sample. Am J Psychiatry 1990;147(5):608–11.

101. De Beurs E, Beekman A, Geerlings S, et al. On becoming depressed or anxious in late life: similar vulnerability factors but different effects of stressful life events. Br J Psychiatry 2001;179(5):426–31.

102. Blazer DG. Depression and social support in late life: a clear but not obvious relationship. Aging Ment Health 2005;9(6):497–9.

103. Chi I, Chou KL. Social support and depression among elderly Chinese people in Hong Kong. Int J Aging Hum Dev 2001;52(3):231–52.

104. Turvey CL, Conwell Y, Jones MP, et al. Risk factors for late-life suicide: a prospective, community-based study. Am J Geriatr Psychiatry 2002;10(4):398–406.

105. Tiikkainen P, Heikkinen RL. Associations between loneliness, depressive symptoms and perceived togetherness in older people. Aging Ment Health 2005;9(6): 526–34.

106. Prince MJ, Harwood RH, Thomas A, et al. A prospective population-based cohort study of the effects of disablement and social milieu on the onset and maintenance of late-life depression. The Gospel Oak Project VII. Psychol Med 1998;28(2):337–50.

107. Chang-Quan H, Zheng-Rong W, Yong-Hong L, et al. Education and risk for late life depression: a meta-analysis of published literature. Int J Psychiatry Med 2010;40(1):109–24.

108. Sexton CE, Mackay CE, Ebmeier KP. A systematic review and meta-analysis of magnetic resonance imaging studies in late-life depression. Am J Geriatr Psychiatry 2013;21(2):184–95.

Cognitive Deficits in Geriatric Depression
Clinical Correlates and Implications for Current and Future Treatment

Sarah Shizuko Morimoto, PsyD*, George S. Alexopoulos, MD

KEYWORDS

- Geriatric depression • Dementia • Cognitive dysfunction • Executive function
- Remission • Cognitive remediation

KEY POINTS

- Major depression in the elderly is often accompanied by cognitive impairment that spans multiple cognitive domains.
- Patients with executive dysfunction are at risk for poor, slow, and unstable antidepressant treatment response, relapse, increased risk of suicidality, and current and future disability.
- MCI emerging during episodes of major late-life depression does not seem to progress to dementia in most cases.
- History of depression is a risk factor that doubles the likelihood of developing dementia in late life.
- In the majority of patients, pharmacologic treatment does not lead to major improvement in cognition, although there are reports that indicate beneficial or deleterious effect on cognition from tricyclics, sertraline, and citalopram.

INTRODUCTION

Major depression in the elderly is often accompanied by cognitive impairment.[1] Although estimates vary, studies have shown that combined depression and cognitive

Funding Sources: Dr S.S. Morimoto, NIMH: K 23 MH 095830, UL1TR00457, The Clinical Translational Science Center at Weill Cornell Medical College; Dr G.S. Alexopoulos, NIMH: P30 MH085943; R01 MH R01 MH096685; R01 MH075897; R01 MH076829; T32 MH019132; The Sanchez Foundation.
Conflicts of Interest: Dr S.S. Morimoto, None; Dr G.S. Alexopoulos, Consultant: Hoffman-LaRoche, Lilly, Pfizer, Otsuka, Speakers' Bureau: Astra Zeneca, Forest, Novartis, Sunovion.
Department of Psychiatry, Institute of Geriatric Psychiatry, Weill Cornell Medical College, 21 Bloomingdale Road, White Plains, NY 10605, USA
* Corresponding author.
E-mail address: ssm9006@med.cornell.edu

Psychiatr Clin N Am 36 (2013) 517–531
http://dx.doi.org/10.1016/j.psc.2013.08.002
0193-953X/13/$ – see front matter © 2013 Elsevier Inc. All rights reserved.

Abbreviations: Cognitive Deficits in Geriatric Depression	
I/P	Initiation/perseveration
DRS	Dementia rating scale
CV/IP	Complex verbal portion of initiation/preservation
DTI	Diffusion tension imaging
ERN	Large error negative wave
Pe	Shallow error positive wave
MCI	Mild cognitive impairment
AD	Alzheimer disease
BDNF	Brain-derived neurotrophic factor
CCR	Computerized cognitive remediation
NBCCR	Neuroplasticity-based computerized cognitive remediation

dysfunction is present in approximately 25% of subjects.[2] In addition, the number of community residents with both depressive symptoms and impaired cognition doubles every 5 years after the age of 70. In some cases, the syndromes of depression and cognitive impairment may be related to the same underlying disorders (eg, vascular dementia and hypothyroidism) whereas, in other cases, depression and cognitive impairment may have different causes but each may influence the course of the other. Differential diagnosis and treatment decisions can be complicated for various reasons. Cognitive symptoms of severe depression can be prominent and be misdiagnosed as an early-stage dementing disorder. Incipient dementia often has somatic and behavioral symptoms resembling depression. Finally, depression is a common complication of dementing disorders.[3] The relationships among cerebrovascular changes, other aging-related structural abnormalities, specific forms of cognitive dysfunction, and increased risk for developing dementias in geriatric depression have yet to be reconciled. The varied and most current findings suggest that there are likely multiple pathways to poor cognitive outcomes.[4]

COGNITIVE DEFICITS IN GERIATRIC DEPRESSION

The neuropsychological impairments seen frequently in geriatric depression span across multiple cognitive domains.[5] These include impairments in

- Episodic memory[6–8]
- Recognition memory
- Visuospatial skills[9–11]
- Verbal fluency[12]
- Psychomotor speed[13,14]

These impairments, in particular memory impairments, were attributed to dysfunction in subcortical structures related to mood regulation, such as the hippocampus.[15]

Recent research has focused on the role of executive functions, such as impaired planning, organizing, initiating, perseverating, sequencing, and attention set shifting in the clinical course of geriatric depression.[9,10,12,16–18] These studies indicate that abnormal performance on some tests of executive function predicts both poor and unstable antidepressant response[12,16,19,20] as well as current and future disability,[21,22] although some disagreement exists.[23] In addition, executive dysfunction has been shown to predict suicidality, even after controlling for comorbid conditions.[24,25] The specifics of this topic are discussed later.

NEUROBIOLOGICAL UNDERPINNINGS OF COGNITIVE DEFICITS

The specific structural and functional abnormalities that contribute to the symptoms of depression remain to be uncovered, although several abnormalities have been reported.[26] Recently, structural and functional neuroimaging have documented both frontostriatal impairment and a relationship between frontostriatal impairment and executive dysfunction in geriatric depression.[27,28]

Structural abnormalities have been identified in the

- Orbitofrontal cortex,[29] particularly in the gyrus rectus bilaterally[30,31]
- Anterior cingulate[30,32]
- Caudate head[33]
- Putamen[34]
- Hippocampus[35,36]
- Amygdala[37]

In addition to gray matter reductions, bilateral white matter hyperintensities are prevalent in geriatric depression[38–41] and mainly occur in the subcortical structures and their frontal projections.[41,42] White matter hyperintensitites disrupt frontostriatal circuits[43] and have been associated with executive dysfunction.[10,27,38]

Abnormal metabolism has also been noted in limbic regions, including the amygdala,[44–46] the pregenual and subgenual anterior cingulate,[47] the posterior orbital cortex,[48] the posterior cingulate, and the medial cerebellum.[49] Recent research has shown increased cortical glucose metabolism in both anterior and posterior cortical regions in patients with geriatric depression relative to controls, particularly in areas where there has been cerebral atrophy, which may represent a compensatory response.[50] Cortical glucose metabolism was correlated with anxiety and depressive symptoms.[50]

Multiple pathways may lead to depression and cognitive impairment. Clinical as well as structural and functional neuroimaging studies suggest, however, that depressive symptoms and executive impairment originate from related brain dysfunctions,[12,20,27,40,51] at least in a subgroup of elderly patients. The authors described a depression–executive dysfunction syndrome, characterized by symptoms and signs resembling a medial frontal lobe syndrome, including psychomotor retardation, anhedonia, apathy, mild vegetative symptoms, and pronounced functional disability disproportional to the severity of the depressive syndrome.[5,16,52]

NEUROCOGNITIVE DEFICITS INFLUENCING TREATMENT RESPONSE OF GERIATRIC DEPRESSION

Abnormal performance on select executive function tests was shown to predict poor and/or slow antidepressant response[12,20,53–55] and a higher level of functional disability.[21]

Select executive functions include processing speed, perseveration, semantic strategy, and response inhibition, which were associated with both poor and unstable antidepressant response and low remission rate in nondemented elderly patients with major depression treated with adequate dosages of various antidepressants.[8,12,16,18–20,26,54–56] Some disagreement exists, however.[23] Dysfunction in the neural circuits related to remission may produce multiple downstream cognitive abnormalities that are similar (ie, semantic strategy deficits vs response inhibition deficits) but not identical, perhaps because of individual differences in network abnormalities, premorbid network characteristics, and network interactions with other brain systems necessary for completion of tasks.[20]

Decrements in performance on the I/P domain of the DRS predict poor response to antidepressant treatment in geriatric depression.[19,57] A meta-analysis examining the relationship between pretreatment cognitive impairment and response to antidepressants demonstrated that only the DRS I/P domain was a reliable predictor of poor antidepressant treatment response.[58] Approximately 42% of elders with major depression have abnormal I/P scores, as measured by the Mattis DRS.[59] Although not a classical test of executive function, the I/P domain of the DRS tests multiple coordinated cognitive skills that require executive functioning. The term, *executive functions*, encompasses a variety of cognitive abilities, such as planning, organizing, self-monitoring, inhibiting prepotent responses, and strategy generation.[60,61] Each of these functions is subserved by distinct, but also shared, neural systems. Furthermore, performance on measures of executive function can affect and be affected by performance in nonexecutive cognitive domains, such as processing speed, learning, and memory.[62]

A recent study showed that among the functions tested by the I/P, only the CV/IP predicted remission during treatment with escitalopram.[12] The CV/IP tests word generation ability by asking patients to name all the items they can think of in a supermarket (ie, semantic fluency). Performance on speeded verbal tasks, such as the CV/IP, can be improved by the use of strategies, such as the organization of responses into superordinate verbal categories (semantic organization) (eg, replying with words belonging to the same category [fruit], such as grapes, strawberries, bananas, and oranges, rather than separate categories, such as bread, bananas, and milk). Completing strategic semantic tasks, such as the CV/IP, also requires selection of words from multiple activated responses and suppression of semantically or phonemically related but inapplicable words. In that study, the use of semantic strategy explained performance differences between remitters and nonremitters.[12]

The authors followed-up these findings with a second study that demonstrated that the use of the same executive function, semantic organizational strategy, explained both verbal memory performance and remission rates of geriatric depression.[20] These studies are the first to define a single executive function that is predictive of remission with antidepressant drug treatment, regardless of the task by which it is elicited. If these findings are replicated, testing semantic strategy use could be an adjunct to a clinical assessment of depressive symptoms to improve clinicians' ability to identify patients at risk for poor antidepressant drug response.[12]

NEUROBIOLOGICAL ABNORMALITIES INFLUENCING TREATMENT RESPONSE OF GERIATRIC DEPRESSION

Structural neuroimaging has documented frontostriatal abnormalities in late-life depression and a relationship of these frontostriatal abnormalities to executive dysfunction.[27,28] A recent study found significant associations between fractional anisotropy in multiple fronto-striato-limbic regions and Stroop color-word interference performance, providing evidence for the association of these areas with the executive dysfunction often accompanying geriatric depression.[27]

Structural abnormalities in neural systems related to executive functions may be associated with poor remission rate of late-life depression. A recent DTI study suggests that reduced white matter integrity in various frontolimbic regions[40,57,63,64] predicts failure to remit with antidepressant treatment in geriatric depression. Older patients with major depression having at least one short allele of the serotonin transporter 5-HTTLPR polymorphism had both microstructural white matter abnormalities in frontolimbic networks and a low remission rate.[65] Similarly, depressed older patients with the $BDNF_{val/val}$ genotype were less likely to achieve remission than $BDNF_{val/met}$ carriers after 12 weeks of treatment with escitalopram (10 mg daily). Unlike carriers of the short 5-HTTLPR allele of the serotonin transporter, however, microstructural abnormalities in the corpus callosum, the left superior corona radiata, and the right inferior longitudinal fasciculus were associated with low remission rate independently of the BDNF allele status.

Studies of brain function identified abnormalities in the cognitive control network that may influence response to antidepressants. Diminished activity in the dorsolateral prefrontal cortex and low functional connectivity between the dorsolateral prefrontal cortex and the dorsal anterior cingulate have been documented in depressed older adults prior to treatment.[28] The authors observed that low resting functional connectivity within a cognitive control network and high functional connectivity within the default mode network characterize late-life major depression.[66] Beyond this double dissociation distinguishing depressed from normal older adults, resting functional connectivity at the cognitive control network, but not connectivity, within the default mode network predicted poor remission rate after treatment with escitalopram and persistence of depression, apathy, and dysexecutive behavior at the end of treatment. In another study, the authors showed that ERN and a Pe after the incongruent conditions of an emotional go-nogo task predicted poor response of major late-life depression to escitalopram; the ERN and Pe are thought to reflect different aspects of conflict processing by the anterior cingulate.[66]

Improvement of depression is often associated with at least partial normalization of abnormal activation of the anterior cingulate[46,63,67–69] and the dorsolateral prefrontal cortex.[28] Greater activation of the rostral and dorsal cingulate at baseline predicts better subsequent antidepressant treatment response[70]; that remission of depression is often associated with at least partial normalization of anterior cingulate activation abnormalities[71,72]; those changes in anterior cingulate function are associated with symptomatic improvement.[73]

THE PROGNOSIS OF DEPRESSION WITH COGNITIVE IMPAIRMENT

MCI during episodes of major late-life depression does not progress to dementia in most cases. Instead, it is a stable disturbance that improves only mildly when depressive symptoms are ameliorated.[26,74,75] Older patients with major depression and a dementia syndrome that subsides after remission of depression (once termed, pseudodementia) are at high risk, however, for developing irreversible dementia.[4,76–79] Taken together, these studies suggest that between 9% and 25% of elderly patients with depression and initially reversible dementia progress into irreversible dementia each year.

Cognitive dysfunction in depressed patients has heterogeneous etiologies and outcomes.[59] Some patients presenting with both cognitive dysfunction and late-onset depression may already have early-stage dementia. This view is supported by findings suggesting that depression is often a prodrome of dementing disorders.[4] As discussed previously, patients with depression and executive dysfunction, have poor and unstable response to antidepressant treatment[12,16,18–20,54–56] and higher risk of relapse as well as poorer social and occupational functioning at follow-up.

DEPRESSION AS A RISK FACTOR AND/OR PRODROME OF DEMENTING DISORDERS

An authoritative meta-analysis of a total sample of more than 100,000 subjects concluded that history of depression doubles the risk for developing dementia in late life.[80] Although the effect sizes of individual studies varied, 19 of the 20 studies used in this meta-analysis yielded a positive relationship between history of depression and risk for developing AD. Examination of the interval between the occurrence of depression and development of dementia suggested that depression is a risk factor for AD rather than a prodrome. This conclusion was consistent with the results of a large study that specifically examined the issue.[81] An earlier study[82] focused on studies that included information on family history of dementia and concluded that a lifetime history of depression increased the risk of AD, regardless of presence or absence of family history of dementing disorders. Severe depression may confer the highest risk for later development of dementia.[83]

In addition to being a risk factor, depressive symptoms are often a prodrome of dementing disorders. In community-residing women, depressive symptoms were associated with poorer cognitive function (Mini-Mental State Examination, Trails B, Digit Symbol) at baseline and with cognitive decline during a 4-year follow-up.[1] Depressed mood at baseline was associated with an increased by 3-fold risk of incident dementia during a 5-year follow-up of elderly community residents.[84] A high prevalence of depressive symptoms and syndromes was observed in individuals with MCI in both hospital-based studies (median: 44.3%) and population-based studies (median: 15.7%). The incidence of depressive symptoms varied from 11.7/100 to 26.6/100 person-years in hospital-based and population-based studies.[85] There is evidence that MCI patients with behavioral features are more prone to developing AD than patients without these features.[86] These findings suggest that depression is both a remote risk factor for dementing disorders and a proximal prodromal feature.[87]

Several pathogenetic mechanisms have been proposed to account for the relationship between depression and risk for dementing disorders. Vascular disease may play a role in the expression of the clinical symptoms of AD, including depressive symptoms. Vascular disease, AD, and depression have common risk factors.[88–90] In addition, inflammatory processes may promote both depression and AD. Some proinflammatory cytokines have been linked to depression, vascular disease, and cognitive compromise[91,92] and the same cytokines may have direct effects on cognitive status particularly in verbal encoding and memory functions.[93] Antidepressants may modify the levels of inflammatory cytokines,[94] but it remains unclear whether antidepressants reduce the risk of AD.

Hypercortesolemia occurring during depressive episodes has been proposed as a factor that may reduce cognitive reserve and promote the expression of cognitive symptoms in patients with dementing disorders. Volumetric studies have found reductions in hippocampal volumes in patients with recurrent major depression.[35,95] Lifetime duration of depression was correlated with hippocampal volume reduction and with behavioral measures of hippocampal function, such as verbal memory.[96] The precise relationship between hypercortisolemia, hippocampal volume loss, and hippocampal inhibitory control is unknown, although animal studies show that neurotoxic tissue damage may be one possible mechanism.

Another possibility may be that excess and chronic secretion of glucocorticoid hormones can reduce neurotrophic factors, inhibit neurogenesis, and render neurons vulnerable to the toxic effect of amyloid. These changes may then compound the neuropathologic changes of AD and accelerate the clinical expression of dementia. The BDNF has been implicated in structural abnormalities of the human hippocampus.[97,98] Several antidepressants elevate BDNF in the rat hippocampus. Recent research suggests that BDNF is rapidly elevated by antidepressant treatments through post-transcriptional mechanisms.[99] Through this action, antidepressants may prevent stress-induced inhibition of neurogenesis and increase dendritic branching.[100] Whether this action delays the onset or inhibits the progression of AD is unclear; systematic studies have not yet explored this question.

CAN THE COGNITIVE DEFICITS OF LATE LIFE DEPRESSION BE MITIGATED WITH DRUG TREATMENT?

Tricyclic antidepressants have not been found to improve cognitive function in depressed older adults. There are some data to suggest they may worsen cognitive functions. Nortriptyline was shown to compromise verbal learning performance of depressed older adults more than placebo.[101] Conversely, some selective serotonin reuptake inhibitors may improve cognitive function mainly in patients whose depressive symptoms subside after treatment. Specifically, sertraline has been shown to improve performance on tests of attention, episodic memory, and executive function[102] but only in treatment responders.[103] Similarly, depressed older patients with an antidepressant response to citalopram showed improvement in psychomotor speed and visuospatial functioning. Conversely, citalopram treatment seemed to have a deleterious effect on neurocognitive functioning in areas of verbal learning and processing speed in patients who remained depressed despite treatment.[104]

A substantial number of depressed older patients continue to experience residual depressive symptoms and neuropsychological deficits after antidepressant treatment. Abnormal executive functions, processing speed, and working memory persist after remission of mood symptoms in many patients with geriatric depression.[28,105,106] In addition, some demographic variables may leave patients more vulnerable to persistent cognitive dysfunction despite treatment: old age, high vascular risk score, and low baseline Mini-Mental State Examination scores all predicted less cognitive improvement in depressed older adults treated with citalopram.[103]

CAN COGNITIVE DEFICITS IN LATE-LIFE DEPRESSION BE MITIGATED WITH COGNITIVE REMEDIATION?

The term, *cognitive remediation*, encompasses a wide variety of interventions. One type of cognitive remediation that the authors think has potential to make clinically relevant change relies on the induction of neuroplasticity (N-CCR) and targets brain networks implicated in late-life depression. Specifically, symptoms and signs of geriatric depression are thought to be mediated by hypometabolism in dorsal neocortical structures, including the dorsolateral prefrontal cortex and differentiation of dorsal anterior cingulate cortex, and hypermetabolism of some limbic structures. In this model, abnormalities underlying executive dysfunction may lead to depression directly by promoting the metabolic changes mediating the depressive syndrome or by serving as conditions predisposing to these metabolic changes.[107] Therefore, in N-CCR interventions designed to treat geriatric depression, the tasks (games) target and activate dorsal neocortical structures in an attempt to enhance their functioning and, therefore, improve signs and symptoms of the depression. Although not all CCR tasks induce neuroplasticity in the aging brain, N-CCR tasks (games) are based on activities that have been shown to activate regions of interest and induce change in the aging brain. To accomplish this goal, N-CCR relies on previous research in induction of neuroplasticity in aging animals to develop principles likely to produce desirable neuroplastic change. N-CCR based on these principles has been applied in treatment trials of aging humans and has demonstrated that structural and functional change is possible given the right training parameters.[50,108,109] Recently, the authors proposed a novel treatment model intended to target and change the functioning of the cerebral networks (discussed previously) through N-CCR.[110]

Pathophysiologic changes leading to executive dysfunction in geriatric depression may be an appropriate target for N-CCR for geriatric depression for at least 3 reasons:

First, the targeted executive deficits seem to rely on related cerebral networks, indicating a possible target for intervention.

Second, the selected executive deficits have a relationship to clinical outcomes.

Third, recent research suggests that CCR based on the principles of neuroplastic reorganization can induce neuroplasticity in the aging brain.[50,111]

Older adults show a training-dependent reduction in diffuse brain activation and increases in specific prefrontal areas, which are correlated with improved performance,[112] perhaps a result of a change in strategic processing. N-CCR targeting executive functions in older adults has been associated with increased resting cerebral blood flow in the prefrontal cortex.[108] Finally, increases in white matter indices (fractional anisotropy and mean diffusivity) in the anterior cingulate cortex and the corpus callosum were observed in DTI studies of older adults who underwent N-CCR training, which correlated with improvements in cognitive performance.[109,113] The authors suggest that directly targeting and changing the function of cerebral network abnormalities that predispose to poor treatment outcomes is a promising strategy likely to produce neurobiological changes leading to a clinically meaningful improvement of depressive symptoms and cognitive outcomes.

Few recent studies have examined whether CCR can improve cognitive deficits in geriatric depression. Based on the observation that patients with geriatric depression exhibit episodic memory impairment, a few studies have been undertaken training memory function in depressed older adults. In these studies, CCR led to improvements in the targeted function (ie, memory) but no effect on depression or other clinical symptoms.[114]

As previously proposed, CCR targeted to clinically relevant cerebral networks may have implications for treating both cognitive and affective symptoms. To the authors' knowledge, there have been no studies implicating memory impairment in the relationship to remission of symptoms. Furthermore, the authors have demonstrated previously that episodic memory impairment in geriatric depression may be at least partially explained by executive dysfunction, specifically the deficient use of verbal strategies.[20] Therefore, that an intervention targeting episodic memory would be unlikely to address both symptom clusters in geriatric depression. More studies of this nature are needed to help demonstrate whether CCR targeted to clinically relevant neural circuitry is necessary to change both cognitive and affective functioning or whether more broad training is sufficient.

SUMMARY

Major depression in the elderly is often accompanied by cognitive impairment[1] and these cognitive deficits span multiple cognitive domains.[5] Certain cognitive deficits have substantial clinical implications, in particular executive dysfunction (ie, susceptibility to interference and semantic strategy). Patients with these deficits are at risk for poor, slow, and unstable antidepressant treatment response; relapse; increased risk of suicidality; and current and future disability. Therefore, it is important that patients exhibiting deficits in executive functions be identified early in treatment so that appropriate treatment planning can be made.

MCI emerging during episodes of major late-life depression does not seem to progress to dementia in most cases. Instead, it is a stable disturbance that improves only mildly when depressive symptoms are ameliorated.[26,74,75] History of depression, however, is a risk factor that doubles the likelihood of developing dementia in late life. In addition, depressive symptoms are often a prodrome of dementing disorders. In theory, depression may be viewed as a modifiable risk factor for AD. This view is intriguing, particularly in light of evidence that antidepressants can reduce the levels of inflammatory cytokines.[94] The possibility that treatment with antidepressants might reduce the risk for AD remains, however, speculative due to the lack of direct studies.

In the majority of patients, pharmacologic treatment does not lead to major improvement in cognition, although there are a few exceptions. There have been reports that tricyclics, such as nortriptyline, may worsen verbal memory more than placebo.[101] Conversely, sertraline and citalopram may improve some cognitive functions but only in those who respond to treatment.[104] In those who do not respond, one study found that citalopram had a deleterious effect on cognition.[115]

Last, novel treatment modalities, such as neuroplasticity-based computerized cognitive remediation, seem to show theoretic promise to produce neurobiological changes and ameliorate affective and cognitive symptoms. More studies are needed in this emerging area.

REFERENCES

1. Yaffe K, Blackwell T, Gore R, et al. Depressive symptoms and cognitive decline in nondemented elderly women: a prospective study. Arch Gen Psychiatry 1999; 56:425–30.
2. Arve S, Tilvis RS, Lehtonen A, et al. Coexistence of lowered mood and cognitive impairment of elderly people in five birth cohorts. Aging (Milano) 1999;11:90–5.
3. Bayles KA, Kazniak AW, et al. Communication and cognition in normal aging and dementia. San Diego (CA): College-Hill Press; 1987.
4. Butters MA, Young JB, Lopez O, et al. Pathways linking late-life depression to persistent cognitive impairment and dementia. Dialogues Clin Neurosci 2008; 10:345–57.
5. Lockwood KA, Alexopoulos GS, van Gorp WG. Executive dysfunction in geriatric depression. Am J Psychiatry 2002;159:1119–26.
6. Beats BC, Sahakian BJ, Levy R. Cognitive performance in tests sensitive to frontal lobe dysfunction in the elderly depressed. Psychol Med 1996;26:591–603.
7. Kramer-Ginsberg E, Greenwald BS, Krishnan KR, et al. Neuropsychological functioning and MRI signal hyperintensities in geriatric depression. Am J Psychiatry 1999;156:438–44.
8. Story TJ, Potter GG, Attix DK, et al. Neurocognitive correlates of response to treatment in late-life depression. Am J Geriatr Psychiatry 2008;16:752–9.
9. Boone KB, Lesser I, Miller B, et al. Cognitive functioning in a mildly to moderately depressed geriatric sample: relationship to chronological age. J Neuropsychiatry Clin Neurosci 1994;6:267–72.
10. Lesser IM, Boone KB, Mehringer CM, et al. Cognition and white matter hyperintensities in older depressed patients. Am J Psychiatry 1996;153:1280–7.
11. Elderkin-Thompson V, Kumar A, Mintz J, et al. Executive dysfunction and visuospatial ability among depressed elders in a community setting. Arch Clin Neuropsychol 2004;19:597–611.
12. Morimoto SS, Gunning FM, Murphy CF, et al. Executive function and short-term remission of geriatric depression: the role of semantic strategy. Am J Geriatr Psychiatry 2011;19:115–22.
13. Butters MA, Whyte EM, Nebes RD, et al. The nature and determinants of neuropsychological functioning in late-life depression. Arch Gen Psychiatry 2004;61: 587–95.
14. Hart RP, Kwentus JA, Taylor JR, et al. Rate of forgetting in dementia and depression. J Consult Clin Psychol 1987;55:101–5.

15. Hickie I, Naismith S, Ward PB, et al. Reduced hippocampal volumes and memory loss in patients with early- and late-onset depression. Br J Psychiatry 2005; 186:197–202.

16. Alexopoulos GS, Meyers BS, Young RC, et al. Executive dysfunction and long-term outcomes of geriatric depression. Arch Gen Psychiatry 2000;57:285–90.

17. Murphy CF, Alexopoulos GS. Longitudinal association of initiation/perseveration and severity of geriatric depression. Am J Geriatr Psychiatry 2004;12:50–6.

18. Potter GG, Kittinger JD, Wagner HR, et al. Prefrontal neuropsychological predictors of treatment remission in late-life depression. Neuropsychopharmacology 2004;29:2266–71.

19. Kalayam B, Alexopoulos GS. Prefrontal dysfunction and treatment response in geriatric depression. Arch Gen Psychiatry 1999;56:713–8.

20. Morimoto SS, Gunning FM, Kanellopoulos D, et al. Semantic organizational strategy predicts verbal memory and remission rate of geriatric depression. Int J Geriatr Psychiatry 2012;27:506–12.

21. Kiosses DN, Klimstra S, Murphy C, et al. Executive dysfunction and disability in elderly patients with major depression. Am J Geriatr Psychiatry 2001;9:269–74.

22. Alexopoulos GS, Kiosses DN, Heo M, et al. Executive dysfunction and the course of geriatric depression. Biol Psychiatry 2005;58:204–10.

23. Butters MA, Bhalla RK, Mulsant BH, et al. Executive functioning, illness course, and relapse/recurrence in continuation and maintenance treatment of late-life depression: is there a relationship? Am J Geriatr Psychiatry 2004;12:387–94.

24. Dombrovski AY, Butters MA, Reynolds CF, et al. Cognitive performance in suicidal depressed elderly: preliminary report. Am J Geriatr Psychiatry 2008;16:109–15.

25. Dombrovski AY, Clark L, Siegle GJ, et al. Reward/Punishment reversal learning in older suicide attempters. Am J Psychiatry 2010;167:699–707.

26. Alexopoulos GS, Kiosses DN, Murphy C, et al. Executive dysfunction, heart disease burden, and remission of geriatric depression. Neuropsychopharmacology 2004;29:2278–84.

27. Murphy CF, Gunning-Dixon FM, Hoptman MJ, et al. White-matter integrity predicts stroop performance in patients with geriatric depression. Biol Psychiatry 2007;61:1007–10.

28. Aizenstein HJ, Butters MA, Wu M, et al. Altered functioning of the executive control circuit in late-life depression: episodic and persistent phenomena. Am J Geriatr Psychiatry 2009;17:30–42.

29. Van Otterloo E, O'Dwyer G, Stockmeier CA, et al. Reductions in neuronal density in elderly depressed are region specific. Int J Geriatr Psychiatry 2009;24:856–64.

30. Ballmaier M, Toga AW, Blanton RE, et al. Anterior cingulate, gyrus rectus, and orbitofrontal abnormalities in elderly depressed patients: an MRI-based parcellation of the prefrontal cortex. Am J Psychiatry 2004;161:99–108.

31. Yuan Y, Zhu W, Zhang Z, et al. Regional gray matter changes are associated with cognitive deficits in remitted geriatric depression: an optimized voxel-based morphometry study. Biol Psychiatry 2008;64:541–4.

32. Drevets WC, Price JL, Simpson JR, et al. Subgenual prefrontal cortex abnormalities in mood disorders. Nature 1997;386:824–7.

33. Krishnan KR, McDonald WM, Escalona PR, et al. Magnetic resonance imaging of the caudate nuclei in depression. Preliminary observations. Arch Gen Psychiatry 1992;49:553–7.

34. Husain MM, McDonald WM, Doraiswamy PM, et al. A magnetic resonance imaging study of putamen nuclei in major depression. Psychiatry Res 1991;40: 95–9.

35. Sheline YI, Wang PW, Gado MH, et al. Hippocampal atrophy in recurrent major depression. Proc Natl Acad Sci U S A 1996;93:3908–13.
36. Lai T, Payne ME, Byrum CE, et al. Reduction of orbital frontal cortex volume in geriatric depression. Biol Psychiatry 2000;48:971–5.
37. Sheline YI, Gado MH, Price JL. Amygdala core nuclei volumes are decreased in recurrent major depression. Neuroreport 1998;9:2023–8.
38. Boone KB, Miller BL, Lesser IM, et al. Neuropsychological correlates of white-matter lesions in healthy elderly subjects. A threshold effect. Arch Neurol 1992;49:549–54.
39. Kumar A, Bilker W, Jin Z, et al. Atrophy and high intensity lesions: complementary neurobiological mechanisms in late-life major depression. Neuropsychopharmacology 2000;22:264–74.
40. Alexopoulos GS, Murphy CF, Gunning-Dixon FM, et al. Microstructural white matter abnormalities and remission of geriatric depression. Am J Psychiatry 2008;165:238–44.
41. Gunning-Dixon FM, Hoptman MJ, Lim KO, et al. Macromolecular white matter abnormalities in geriatric depression: a magnetization transfer imaging study. Am J Geriatr Psychiatry 2008;16:255–62.
42. MacFall JR, Payne ME, Provenzale JE, et al. Medial orbital frontal lesions in late-onset depression. Biol Psychiatry 2001;49:803–6.
43. Hannestad J, Taylor WD, McQuoid DR, et al. White matter lesion volumes and caudate volumes in late-life depression. Int J Geriatr Psychiatry 2006;21:1193–8.
44. Wu JC, Gillin JC, Buchsbaum MS, et al. Effect of sleep deprivation on brain metabolism of depressed patients. Am J Psychiatry 1992;149:538–43.
45. Drevets WC. Prefrontal cortical-amygdalar metabolism in major depression. Ann N Y Acad Sci 1999;877:614–37.
46. Drevets WC, Bogers W, Raichle ME. Functional anatomical correlates of antidepressant drug treatment assessed using PET measures of regional glucose metabolism. Eur Neuropsychopharmacol 2002;12:527–44.
47. Drevets WC. Functional neuroimaging studies of depression: the anatomy of melancholia. Annu Rev Med 1998;49:341–61.
48. Drevets WC, Videen TO, Price JL, et al. A functional anatomical study of unipolar depression. J Neurosci 1992;12:3628–41.
49. Bench CJ, Friston KJ, Brown RG, et al. The anatomy of melancholia–focal abnormalities of cerebral blood flow in major depression. Psychol Med 1992;22:607–15.
50. Smith GE, Housen P, Yaffe K, et al. A cognitive training program based on principles of brain plasticity: results from the Improvement in Memory with Plasticity-based Adaptive Cognitive Training (IMPACT) study. J Am Geriatr Soc 2009;57:594–603.
51. Alexopoulos GS, Katz IR, Reynolds CF, et al. Depression in older adults. J Psychiatr Pract 2001;7:441–6.
52. Alexopoulos GS, Vrontou C, Kakuma T, et al. Disability in geriatric depression. Am J Psychiatry 1996;153:877–85.
53. Alexopoulos GS, Kiosses DN, Choi SJ, et al. Frontal white matter microstructure and treatment response of late-life depression: a preliminary study. Am J Psychiatry 2002;159:1929–32.
54. Sneed JR, Roose SP, Keilp JG, et al. Response inhibition predicts poor antidepressant treatment response in very old depressed patients. Am J Geriatr Psychiatry 2007;15:553–63.

55. Sneed JR, Keilp JG, Brickman AM, et al. The specificity of neuropsychological impairment in predicting antidepressant non-response in the very old depressed. Int J Geriatr Psychiatry 2008;23:319–23.

56. Simpson S, Baldwin RC, Jackson A, et al. Is subcortical disease associated with a poor response to antidepressants? Neurological, neuropsychological and neuroradiological findings in late-life depression. Psychol Med 1998;28: 1015–26.

57. Alexopoulos GS. Role of executive function in late-life depression. J Clin Psychiatry 2003;64(Suppl 14):18–23.

58. McLennan SN, Mathias JL. The depression-executive dysfunction (DED) syndrome and response to antidepressants: a meta-analytic review. Int J Geriatr Psychiatry 2010;25:933–44.

59. Alexopoulos GS, Kiosses DN, Klimstra S, et al. Clinical presentation of the "depression-executive dysfunction syndrome" of late life. Am J Geriatr Psychiatry 2002;10:98–106.

60. Lezak MD. Neuropsychological assessment. New York: Oxford University Press; 1976.

61. Benton AL. Contributions to neuropsychological assessment: a clinical manual. 2nd edition. New York: Oxford University Press; 1994.

62. Elderkin-Thompson V, Hellemann G, Pham D, et al. Prefrontal brain morphology and executive function in healthy and depressed elderly. Int J Geriatr Psychiatry 2009;24:459–68.

63. Kennedy SH, Evans KR, Krüger S, et al. Changes in regional brain glucose metabolism measured with positron emission tomography after paroxetine treatment of major depression. Am J Psychiatry 2001;158:899–905.

64. Alexopoulos GS, Glatt CE, Hoptman MJ, et al. BDNF val66met polymorphism, white matter abnormalities and remission of geriatric depression. J Affect Disord 2010;125:262–8.

65. Alexopoulos GS, Murphy CF, Gunning-Dixon FM, et al. Serotonin transporter polymorphisms, microstructural white matter abnormalities and remission of geriatric depression. J Affect Disord 2009;119:132–41.

66. Alexopoulos GS, Hoptman MJ, Kanellopoulos D, et al. Functional connectivity in the cognitive control network and the default mode network in late-life depression. J Affect Disord 2012;139:56–65.

67. Buchsbaum MS, Wu J, Siegel BV, et al. Effect of sertraline on regional metabolic rate in patients with affective disorder. Biol Psychiatry 1997;41:15–22.

68. Saxena S, Brody AL, Ho ML, et al. Differential cerebral metabolic changes with paroxetine treatment of obsessive-compulsive disorder vs major depression. Arch Gen Psychiatry 2002;59:250–61.

69. Gildengers AG, Houck PR, Mulsant BH, et al. Trajectories of treatment response in late-life depression: psychosocial and clinical correlates. J Clin Psychopharmacol 2005;25:S8–13.

70. Langenecker SA, Kennedy SE, Guidotti LM, et al. Frontal and limbic activation during inhibitory control predicts treatment response in major depressive disorder. Biol Psychiatry 2007;62:1272–80.

71. Mayberg HS, Liotti M, Brannan SK, et al. Reciprocal limbic-cortical function and negative mood: converging PET findings in depression and normal sadness. Am J Psychiatry 1999;156:675–82.

72. Wu J, Buchsbaum MS, Gillin JC, et al. Prediction of antidepressant effects of sleep deprivation by metabolic rates in the ventral anterior cingulate and medial prefrontal cortex. Am J Psychiatry 1999;156:1149–58.

73. Fu CH, Williams SC, Cleare AJ, et al. Attenuation of the neural response to sad faces in major depression by antidepressant treatment: a prospective, event-related functional magnetic resonance imaging study. Arch Gen Psychiatry 2004;61:877–89.

74. Murphy CF, Alexopoulos GS. Attention network dysfunction and treatment response of geriatric depression. J Clin Exp Neuropsychol 2006;28:96–100.

75. Nakano Y, Baba H, Maeshima H, et al. Executive dysfunction in medicated, remitted state of major depression. J Affect Disord 2008;111:46–51.

76. Reynolds CF, Kupfer DJ, Hoch CC, et al. Two-year follow-up of elderly patients with mixed depression and dementia. Clinical and electroencephalographic sleep findings. J Am Geriatr Soc 1986;34:793–9.

77. Kral VA, Emery OB. Long-term follow-up of depressive pseudodementia of the aged. Can J Psychiatry 1989;34:445–6.

78. Copeland JR, Davidson IA, Dewey ME, et al. Alzheimer's disease, other dementias, depression and pseudodementia: prevalence, incidence and three-year outcome in Liverpool. Br J Psychiatry 1992;161:230–9.

79. Alexopoulos GS, Meyers BS, Young RC, et al. The course of geriatric depression with "reversible dementia": a controlled study. Am J Psychiatry 1993;150: 1693–9.

80. Ownby RL, Crocco E, Acevedo A, et al. Depression and risk for Alzheimer disease: systematic review, meta-analysis, and metaregression analysis. Arch Gen Psychiatry 2006;63:530–8.

81. Green RC, Cupples LA, Kurz A, et al. Depression as a risk factor for Alzheimer disease: the MIRAGE Study. Arch Neurol 2003;60:753–9.

82. van Duijn CM, Hendriks L, Farrer LA, et al. A population-based study of familial Alzheimer disease: linkage to chromosomes 14, 19, and 21. Am J Hum Genet 1994;55:714–27.

83. Chen R, Hu Z, Wei L, et al. Severity of depression and risk for subsequent dementia: cohort studies in China and the UK. Br J Psychiatry 2008;193: 373–7.

84. Devanand DP, Sano M, Tang MX, et al. Depressed mood and the incidence of Alzheimer's disease in the elderly living in the community. Arch Gen Psychiatry 1996;53:175–82.

85. Panza F, Frisardi V, Capurso C, et al. Late-life depression, mild cognitive impairment, and dementia: possible continuum? Am J Geriatr Psychiatry 2010;18: 98–116.

86. Apostolova LG, Cummings JL. Neuropsychiatric manifestations in mild cognitive impairment: a systematic review of the literature. Dement Geriatr Cogn Disord 2008;25:115–26.

87. Alexopoulos GS, Buckwalter K, Olin J, et al. Comorbidity of late life depression: an opportunity for research on mechanisms and treatment. Biol Psychiatry 2002; 52:543–58.

88. Alexopoulos GS. The vascular depression hypothesis: 10 years later. Biol Psychiatry 2006;60:1304–5.

89. Iadecola C, Gorelick PB. Converging pathogenic mechanisms in vascular and neurodegenerative dementia. Stroke 2003;34:335–7.

90. Rasgon N, Jarvik L. Insulin resistance, affective disorders, and Alzheimer's disease: review and hypothesis. J Gerontol A Biol Sci Med Sci 2004;59:178–83 [discussion: 184–92].

91. Alexopoulos GS, Morimoto SS. The inflammation hypothesis in geriatric depression. Int J Geriatr Psychiatry 2011;26:1109–18.

92. Morimoto SS, Alexopoulos GS. Immunity, aging, and geriatric depression. Psychiatr Clin North Am 2011;34:437–49, ix.
93. Elderkin-Thompson V, Irwin MR, Hellemann G, et al. Interleukin-6 and memory functions of encoding and recall in healthy and depressed elderly adults. Am J Geriatr Psychiatry 2012;20:753–63.
94. Castanon N, Leonard BE, Neveu PJ, et al. Effects of antidepressants on cytokine production and actions. Brain Behav Immun 2002;16:569–74.
95. Sheline YI, Gado MH, Kraemer HC. Untreated depression and hippocampal volume loss. Am J Psychiatry 2003;160:1516–8.
96. Sheline YI, Sanghavi M, Mintun MA, et al. Depression duration but not age predicts hippocampal volume loss in medically healthy women with recurrent major depression. J Neurosci 1999;19:5034–43.
97. Pezawas L, Verchinski BA, Mattay VS, et al. The brain-derived neurotrophic factor val66met polymorphism and variation in human cortical morphology. J Neurosci 2004;24:10099–102.
98. Bueller JA, Aftab M, Sen S, et al. BDNF Val66Met allele is associated with reduced hippocampal volume in healthy subjects. Biol Psychiatry 2006;59: 812–5.
99. Musazzi L, Cattaneo A, Tardito D, et al. Early raise of BDNF in hippocampus suggests induction of posttranscriptional mechanisms by antidepressants. BMC Neurosci 2009;10:48.
100. Duman RS, Heninger GR, Nestler EJ. A molecular and cellular theory of depression. Arch Gen Psychiatry 1997;54:597–606.
101. Meyers BS, Mattis S, Gabriele M, et al. Effects of nortriptyline on memory self-assessment and performance in recovered elderly depressives. Psychopharmacol Bull 1991;27:295–9.
102. Barch DM, D'Angelo G, Pieper C, et al. Cognitive improvement following treatment in late-life depression: relationship to vascular risk and age of onset. Am J Geriatr Psychiatry 2012;20:682–90.
103. Devanand DP, Pelton GH, Marston K, et al. Sertraline treatment of elderly patients with depression and cognitive impairment. Int J Geriatr Psychiatry 2003; 18:123–30.
104. Culang ME, Sneed JR, Keilp JG, et al. Change in cognitive functioning following acute antidepressant treatment in late-life depression. Am J Geriatr Psychiatry 2009;17:881–8.
105. Nebes RD, Pollock BG, Houck PR, et al. Persistence of cognitive impairment in geriatric patients following antidepressant treatment: a randomized, double-blind clinical trial with nortriptyline and paroxetine. J Psychiatr Res 2003;37: 99–108.
106. Butters MA, Becker JT, Nebes RD, et al. Changes in cognitive functioning following treatment of late-life depression. Am J Psychiatry 2000;157:1949–54.
107. Alexopoulos GS. Depression in the elderly. Lancet 2005;365:1961–70.
108. Mozolic JL, Hayasaka S, Laurienti PJ. A cognitive training intervention increases resting cerebral blood flow in healthy older adults. Front Hum Neurosci 2010;4:16.
109. Lovden M, Bodammer NC, Kuhn S, et al. Experience-dependent plasticity of white-matter microstructure extends into old age. Neuropsychologia 2010;48: 3878–83.
110. Morimoto SS, Wexler BE, Alexopoulos GS. Neuroplasticity-based computerized cognitive remediation for geriatric depression. Int J Geriatr Psychiatry 2012;27: 1239–47.

111. Mahncke HW, Connor BB, Appelman J, et al. Memory enhancement in healthy older adults using a brain plasticity-based training program: a randomized, controlled study. Proc Natl Acad Sci U S A 2006;103:12523–8.

112. Erickson KI, Colcombe SJ, Wadhwa R, et al. Training-induced plasticity in older adults: effects of training on hemispheric asymmetry. Neurobiol Aging 2007;28: 272–83.

113. Takeuchi H, Sekiguchi A, Taki Y, et al. Training of working memory impacts structural connectivity. J Neurosci 2010;30:3297–303.

114. Naismith SL, Redoblado-Hodge MA, Lewis SJ, et al. Cognitive training in affective disorders improves memory: a preliminary study using the NEAR approach. J Affect Disord 2010;121:258–62.

115. Sneed JR, Culang ME, Keilp JG, et al. Antidepressant medication and executive dysfunction: a deleterious interaction in late-life depression. Am J Geriatr Psychiatry 2010;18:128–35.

The Two-Way Relationship Between Medical Illness and Late-Life Depression

Ondria C. Gleason, MD*, Aaron M. Pierce, DO,
Ashley E. Walker, MD, Julia K. Warnock, MD

KEYWORDS

- Comorbidities • Late-life depression • Late-life physical health

KEY POINTS

- The cause-and-effect relationship between depression and physical health remains ill-defined, although the association between them is apparent.
- Clinicians are challenged to make accurate diagnoses and prescribe safe and effective treatment for elderly patients with mental and medical comorbidities.
- Adverse effects of prescribed medications, alcohol, or other substance use and other physical and environmental factors may play a role in the patient's outcome.

INTRODUCTION

Medical illness is common in the geriatric population. Psychiatric conditions are also prevalent, with depression being the most common mental health problem experienced by older individuals. In many cases, the presence of either depression or medical illness increases the incidence of the other. Furthermore, depression that is comorbid with another medical illness predicts a worse medical outcome. This 2-way relationship is of increasing interest as the population ages and as the etiology of depression continues to elude science, while it becomes increasingly apparent that a complex interaction between biologic and environmental factors is involved. Nemeroff and Owens[1] summarized our current understanding of the biologic underpinnings of depression and categorized this into 3 general systems of altered function: the vascular system, the monoamine neurotransmitter systems, and alterations in the hypothalamic-pituitary-adrenal (HPA) axis. These systems are also involved in many common medical conditions.

The association between depression and general medical conditions is multifaceted. Symptoms of depression often overlap with symptoms of general medical

Department of Psychiatry, The University of Oklahoma School of Community Medicine, 4502 East 41st Street, Tulsa, OK 74135-2512, USA
* Corresponding author.
E-mail address: Ondria-gleason@ouhsc.edu

Psychiatr Clin N Am 36 (2013) 533–544
http://dx.doi.org/10.1016/j.psc.2013.08.003
0193-953X/13/$ – see front matter © 2013 Elsevier Inc. All rights reserved.

Abbreviations: Medical Illness and Late-Life Depression	
HPA	Hypothalamic-pituitary-adrenal
AMI	Acute myocardial infarction
MDD	Major depressive disorder
PCP	Primary care physician
SSRIs	Selective serotonin reuptake inhibitors
TCAs	Tricyclic antidepressants
TSH	Thyroid-stimulating hormone
DHEAS	Dehydroepiandrosterone sulfate
HPG	Hypothalamic-pituitary-gonadal
COPD	Chronic obstructive pulmonary disease
ESRD	End-stage renal disease
CKD	Chronic kidney disease
HCV	Hepatitis C virus

conditions, and the order of onset is often difficult to determine, making the diagnostic process even more difficult. Depression often coexists with general medical conditions, such as cardiovascular and endocrine problems, as well as pulmonary, kidney, and gastrointestinal diseases. The presence of multiple conditions further complicates treatment, as does associated medication use, substance abuse problems (often underappreciated in the elderly), age-related changes in sleep architecture, and an array of other psychosocial and environmental factors that can contribute to the development of depression (**Box 1**, **Table 1**). This article reviews some common medical conditions and the interaction between those illnesses and depression in the geriatric population. We aim to help clarify the 2-way interaction between depression and these medical conditions, especially in older individuals, and hope to impart some important diagnostic and treatment considerations to the practicing physician.

LATE-LIFE DEPRESSION AND CARDIOVASCULAR DISEASE

Since the 1970s, studies have delineated a link between depression and cardiovascular disease, and mortality. Even after controlling for potential confounders, such as age, smoking, and other behavioral and medical factors, depression confers an increased risk for developing ischemic heart disease (by 1.5-fold to 2.0-fold), as well as dying from cardiac disease.[2,3] Depressive symptoms have consistently been shown to predict adverse outcomes and hospital readmission, increase the frequency of cardiac events (independent of other risk factors), and negatively impact the

Box 1	
Psychosocial factors relevant to geriatric depression	
Bereavement	Hearing loss
Loss of independence	Vision loss
Transportation	Housing
Retirement	Distance from family
Isolation	Ageism
Loss of function	Elder abuse
Financial	

Table 1
Classes of drugs that may cause depression symptoms

Drug Class	Examples
Angiotension-converting enzyme inhibitors	Captopril, enalapril, lisinopril
Antibiotics	Ciprofloxacin, cycloserine, dapsone, metronidazole, trimethoprim-sulfamethoxazole
Anticholinergics	Dicyclomine, scopolamine
Antivirals	Acyclovir, efavirenz, interferon alfa, nevirapine
Barbiturates	Phenobarbital, secobarbital
Benzodiazepines	Alprazolam, chlordiazepoxide, clonazepam, diazepam, lorazepam, temazepam, triazolam
Calcium-channel blockers	Diltiazem, nifedipine, verapamil
Corticosteroids	Prednisone, cortisone, adrenocorticotropic hormone
Dermatologics	Finasteride, isotretinoin
H_2-antihistamines	Cimetidine, famotidine, nizatidine, ranitidine
Nonsteroidal anti-inflammatory drugs	Ibuprofen, indomethacin, naproxen, meloxicam
Opioids	Codeine, meperidine, morphine, oxycodone
Parkinson drugs	Amantadine, levodopa, pramipexole, ropinirole

functional benefits from coronary artery bypass graft surgery. The impact may be even greater in women than in men, for unclear reasons.[4]

Studies also indicate that 16% to 18% of patients in the hospital after an acute myocardial infarction (AMI) are affected by major depression, and a total of about one-third will experience depression at some point during the first year after the AMI, especially in the first 6 months afterward.[5] Major depressive disorder (MDD) has been reported to increase mortality by 3.5-fold in the first 6 months following an AMI, and 2.0-fold over 6.7 years of follow-up. Independent factors associated with this doubling of long-term mortality rate include severity of MDD and failure of depression to improve substantially within 6 months of treatment.[6]

An estimated 15% to 23% of those with established ischemic heart disease may have MDD, and depression in this population conveys a three-fold to four-fold increase in subsequent cardiovascular morbidity and mortality.[7] In the Cardiovascular Health Study, a large population-based study of persons 65 and older, approximately 20% met the cutoff score for clinical depression, and these people were more likely to die in the follow-up period (average of 6 years), as were those with milder or subthreshold forms of depression. Those with high depression scores had mortality risks 25% to 43% higher than those with low depression scores; hypertension, congestive heart failure, or stroke all also increased the risk of dying.[8] The Rotterdam Study, a population-based cohort study, found that subjects age 60 years and older with atherosclerosis were more likely to be depressed, and more severe atherosclerosis correlated with higher depression rating scores.[9]

The past decade has provided increasing evidence for a "vascular depression," which may be more common with late-onset as opposed to early-onset depression in late life. It has also been described as a "depression-executive dysfunction syndrome" and may have a different clinical presentation from other major depression, characterized by psychomotor retardation, greater anhedonia, impaired verbal fluency and visual naming, and poor performance on tasks of initiation and perseverance. It is also associated with less family history, greater functional disability, and perhaps worse treatment outcomes.[10]

Although the exact relationship remains unclear, vascular disease may contribute to late-life depression by affecting subcortical structures involved in mood regulation and the white matter pathways that connect these structures to the frontal cortex.[11] Although this may seem related more to cerebrovascular disease, there is clearly a relation to cardiovascular disease. Physiologic changes that could contribute to adverse cardiac results include immune or inflammatory activation, decreased myocardial perfusion, elevated catecholamines, platelet aggregation, impairment of arterial endothelial functioning, cardiac arrhythmia, increased sympathetic tone, hypercortisolemia, abnormal folate or homocysteine metabolism, and reduced heart rate variability.[9,12–14] Atherosclerosis, genetic risk factors, and stress may also represent a shared underlying etiology of depression and vascular disease; increased activity by anti-inflammatory enzyme 5-lipoxygenase has been proposed as a common mechanism for atherosclerosis and depression.[15] Nonbiological factors, too, clearly play a role in depression and cardiovascular outcomes; depressed patients are significantly less likely to adhere to prescribed medications, follow lifestyle recommendations (eg, smoking cessation, exercise), practice self-management (eg, monitor weight and adjust diuretics in heart failure), and follow-up with or receive recommended cardiac testing.

CLINICAL VIGNETTE: LATE-LIFE DEPRESSION AND HEART DISEASE

Mr A is a 66-year-old White man with no prior psychiatric history who presents to his primary care physician (PCP) 3 months after having a heart attack with stent placement. He reports 2 months of poor sleep, decreased motivation, spending more time in his room, and low energy. He denies feeling sad but does feel more anxious than before. He has not followed the PCP's recommendations on diet, smoking, or exercise, but has still lost about 5 pounds since he was last seen. He wants to know what is going on and what his PCP recommends for treatment.

Mr A endorses many symptoms of late-life depression, which may present somewhat differently from depression in younger patients, and is also within the post-MI window during which he is at increased risk of mortality. He and his family should be counseled on depression in the setting of cardiovascular disease and treatment options, including psychotherapy or pharmacotherapy. Preferred medications for treatment of depression with comorbid cardiovascular disease are selective serotonin reuptake inhibitors (SSRIs) and venlafaxine, because of their favorable side-effect profiles. Of the SSRIs, sertraline and citalopram in particular have been shown in trials to be safe and effective for patients with coronary heart disease (CHD) and depression.[14] Tricyclic antidepressants (TCAs) should be avoided if possible because of potential weight gain, increased QT interval, risk of torsades de pointes, and orthostatic hypotension.[3,7,16]

Care should be taken in administering SSRIs concomitantly with certain cardiac medications, because of cytochrome P450 enzyme interactions. For example, fluvoxamine inhibits CYP 1A and CYP 2C. Paroxetine and fluoxetine inhibit CYP 2D6 and CYP 3A4, leading to increased concentration of any cardiac drugs also metabolized by these enzymes. Sertraline and venlafaxine also inhibit CYP2D6, although to a lesser degree. Other notable cardiovascular effects of antidepressants include tachycardia and hypertension with venlafaxine, and QT prolongation in citalopram overdose.[15] Up to 25% of patients stop their antidepressants during the first 6 months of treatment because of adverse effects or lack of efficacy, so potential interactions and effects should be closely monitored.[14]

Cognitive behavioral therapy is a viable alternative for patients who cannot tolerate antidepressants or prefer nonpharmacologic treatment, and may also be used in conjunction with an antidepressant. Cardiac rehabilitation and aerobic exercise, if appropriate for the individual, can also improve both depression and cardiovascular health. Clinically significant depression should not be viewed as a "normal" reaction that will remit after the stress of an acute cardiac event.[14] It must be aggressively screened for, appropriately evaluated and treated, and carefully monitored in the high-risk setting of cardiovascular disease.

LATE-LIFE DEPRESSION AND ENDOCRINE DISORDERS

When considering changes in endocrine function in an older person with major depression, it can be difficult to differentiate the effects of aging on endocrine physiology from those caused by another age-related illness. Psychiatrists are generally judicious about examining patients for thyroid endocrinopathies, and any pathology along the hypothalamic-pituitary-thyroid axis is generally ascertained through appropriate laboratory testing. However, one aging effect is an increased level of thyroid-stimulating hormone, particularly in postmenopausal women. Studies indicate that age-related cases of subclinical hypothyroidism can potentially be as high as 23%.[17] One of many conundrums when assessing late-life depression is to determine when the changes of an aging thyroid become significant to the point of exacerbating or manifesting as symptoms of depression in an older person.

Perhaps an understudied area of late-life depression involves age-related decreases in ovarian and testicular function. Some symptoms of depression in later life may be bidirectional, with age-related endocrine changes, such as low testosterone or estrogen. Unlike menopause, when estrogen deficiency is associated with known clinical consequences, the decline in androgens in aging men varies from modest to severe, but with unclear clinical consequences. However, more than 70% of men older than 70 years have free testosterone levels consistent with hypogonadism.[18] Decreased levels of testosterone in men are associated with depression, fatigue, hot flushes, sweating, and weight gain.[19] Hypogonadal levels of testosterone are also associated with decline in muscle mass, increase in fat mass, decreased muscle strength, anemia, and decreased bone mineral density.

In addition to age-related decline in testosterone, the chronic use of substances such as alcohol and opioids may raise additional concern about adverse effects on patients' pituitary-hypothalamic-gonadal (HPG) function. Abuse of alcohol is common and underrecognized in the elderly, as is the use of opioids in the management of chronic pain. Adverse consequences of both alcohol and opioids include fatigue, depression, and sexual dysfunction.

Chronic use of substances such as alcohol and opioids can decrease levels of the gonadal sex hormones, testosterone, and estrogens. Opioids, in particular, are known to decrease growth hormone, cortisol, and dehydroepiandrosterone sulfate. This now well-described syndrome of decreased gonadal and adrenal androgen production is called opioid-induced endocrinopathy.[20,21] It is estimated that the number of men in the United States and Canada treated with sustained-action opioids is more than 5 million. Investigators report that a substantial proportion of these individuals on opioids are testosterone deficient.[22] It is common for medical conditions and substance use issues to complicate the assessment of patients with late-life depression, as demonstrated in the following case.

CLINICAL VIGNETTE: LATE-LIFE DEPRESSION AND ENDOCRINE DISEASE (LOW TESTOSTERONE)

Mr B is a 65-year-old married white male with a depressed mood for the past decade who was referred for psychiatric evaluation and treatment. He had 1 prior psychiatric hospitalization 5 years previously for depression with suicidal ideation. At that time, he was also heavily drinking alcohol, retrospectively recognizing it as a means to self-treat his depression. Following the hospitalization, he remained abstinent from alcohol with the help of Alcoholics Anonymous, although his depression remained. He saw 5 different psychiatrists and had been treated with fluoxetine, fluvoxamine, desipramine, nefazodone, bupropion, and venlafaxine. He denied effectiveness of any of these treatments. Attempted augmentation with lithium led to an "out-of-body experience," so lithium was discontinued. Thyroid augmentation had also been attempted without benefit. During that time, he was also diagnosed with attention-deficit hyperactivity disorder and was treated with methylpheni-date and d-amphetamine and l-amphetamine salts. Again, there was no symptom relief and he worried that he would become a "pill head."

His presenting depressive symptoms included melancholy with agitation, impaired concentra-tion, and feelings of worthlessness. The antidepressant, escitalopram, was started without benefit. His testosterone level was obtained, revealing a low level of 247 ng/dL (normal range 270 to 1070 ng/dL). He was started on sertraline in combination with testosterone (150 mg intra-muscularly monthly) and reported, "I think we're on the right track," after a month of treat-ment. Three months later, he reported, "I've been doing great." And, approximately 10 months after beginning testosterone, his depression was in full remission. A few months later, however, Mr B lost his job and his insurance would no longer cover the testosterone. Within a month, his depression completely relapsed with early morning awakening and feel-ings of worthlessness. A recheck of his testosterone level showed it to be 208 ng/dL. His testos-terone treatments were reinitiated and 2 months later, his depression had lifted and he reported, "This is the best that I've been in years."

Mr B appears to have suffered from major depression, severe, in combination with a probable substance-induced endocrinopathy due to his chronic alcohol abuse. Management of Mr B's very resistant depression required testosterone supplementation in addition to antidepressant therapy. With the increase in alcohol abuse and opioid use in older people, substance-induced endocrinopathies are important considerations in the assessment and treatment of late-life depression.

It is also known that in depressed men and women, the HPA axis activity is increased, while ac-tivity of the HPG axis is diminished. The increase in HPA axis activity results in high levels of cu-mulative glucocorticosteroid exposure, resulting in neuronal damage that selectively affects hippocampal structure and inflammatory pathways.[23] Certainly some individuals with these ab-normalities will present to the psychiatrist's office with difficult-to-treat psychiatric and medical symptoms.

LATE-LIFE DEPRESSION AND CHRONIC OBSTRUCTIVE PULMONARY DISEASE

Chronic obstructive pulmonary disease (COPD), which includes 2 main conditions, chronic bronchitis and emphysema, is characterized by airflow limitation that is not fully reversible. COPD is usually diagnosed in middle or old age and affects more than 24 million adults in the United States.[24] Depression frequently co-occurs with COPD, with prevalence of comorbid depression varying from 10% to 42%, with the highest rates of depression in those who are oxygen dependent.[25,26]

Struggles with loss of independence, inability to carry out previous activities, and social isolation may play a role in the depression these patients experience and many patients have temporary depressive symptoms during COPD-related exacerba-tions that resolve once their respiratory symptoms improve. However, comorbid depression is associated with poorer physical functioning, lower treatment adherence, increased hospitalizations, and mortality, and is found to predict fatigue, shortness of breath, and disability in those with COPD, even after adjusting for severity of illness.[25] More than 80% of COPD cases are associated with smoking, and smokers are more likely to either restart smoking or smoke more heavily during periods of distress, which in turn may worsen respiratory status. Increased use of alcohol by depressed patients with COPD may put such patients at increased risk of severe community-acquired pneumonia, particularly aspiration pneumonia.[27–30]

Awareness of the effects that medications used for depression and COPD have on each illness must be maintained. Corticosteroids used in the treatment of COPD may cause depressive symptoms.[31] Oral theophyllines, which are adenosine-receptor an-tagonists, may disrupt sleep in depressed patients with COPD.[32] Difficulties with sleep are common in COPD and depression; benzodiazepines must be used cautiously in this population, as they may reduce the ventilatory response to hypoxia.

Depression in COPD may go undiagnosed because of the limited awareness (by both patients and providers) of this comorbidity; limited skills, time, and resources during provider visits; and misattribution of depressive symptoms as symptoms of COPD.[33] Many symptoms of depression and COPD may overlap and care must be taken to avoid mistaking symptoms of worsening COPD for depression and vice versa, but sustained depressed mood or anhedonia should not be attributed to lung disease alone.[25] Loss of energy, poor memory and concentration, weight loss, and sleep disturbances can be common symptoms in either depression or COPD.

LATE-LIFE DEPRESSION AND CHRONIC RENAL DISEASE

Depression is the most common psychiatric disorder found in patients with end-stage renal disease (ESRD). A study of patients with chronic kidney disease (CKD) stages 2 to 5, with a mean age of 64.5 years, demonstrated a prevalence of major depression to be 21%, which did not vary significantly between stages.[34] Depression has been associated with poorer outcomes, such as death and hospitalization in patients receiving dialysis, even after controlling for age, sex, race, time on dialysis, and other medical comorbidities; suicide rates may be 15 times higher than in the general population.[35,36] The diagnosis of depression in patients with CKD can be complicated, as many of the symptoms seen in CKD, such as poor concentration, anergia, loss of appetite, disrupted sleep, and decreased libido, are also common symptoms of depression. The diagnosis of depression in patients with CKD may be better indicated by feelings of helplessness, hopelessness, and worthlessness, and thoughts of suicide.[37] Although functional decline, diminished independence, changes in roles and responsibilities, and limitations imposed by dialysis treatment may all play a role in depression in patients with CKD, the hypersecretion of proinflammatory cytokines in CKD may also play a role via malfunction of noradrenergic and serotonergic neurotransmission in the brain and endocrinological abnormalities, such as hyperparathyroidism.[38,39]

The effects of depression itself may have a negative impact on the course of CKD; for example, decreased oral intake related to depression may worsen the anemia and malnutrition common in patients receiving hemodialysis.[38] Additionally, depression seems to be a significant risk factor for noncompliance in patients with chronic medical conditions and this relationship may be even stronger in patients with ESRD; noncompliance in patients receiving chronic hemodialysis has been associated with increased mortality.[40,41] The negative effects of depression on positive expectations for improvement, maintenance of strong social support, and cognitive functioning all may be factors in affecting adherence in these patients.[40] Depression should be considered an important modifiable risk factor for outcomes for these patients.[42]

LATE-LIFE DEPRESSION AND GASTROINTESTINAL DISEASE

There is a close relationship between the gut and the brain, resulting in frequently co-occurring gastrointestinal disorders and psychiatric disorders. Physiologic changes associated with aging, environmental factors such as smoking, and use of nonsteroidal anti-inflammatory drugs and other medications increase the risk of gastrointestinal disorders, especially those related to acid production, in the elderly.[43] Gastroenterologists distinguish between "functional" and "structural" gastrointestinal disorders. Functional disorders include irritable bowel syndrome and functional dyspepsia, whereas structural disorders are those in which a specific lesion or lesions can be identified or visualized. Clinical epidemiologic studies have shown that approximately 50% of patients with "functional" disorders have comorbid mood or anxiety disorders, compared with 15% to 30% of patients with "structural" disorders.[44] Interestingly, the onset of both anxiety and depression tend to occur at approximately the same time as the onset of the irritable bowel syndrome, suggesting a potentially common etiologic pathway.

Anxiety disorders are common among patients with gastrointestinal disorders in general, although depression tends to be seen in patients with more chronic, unremitting illness.[45] The presence of psychiatric illness, including depression, predicts a poorer prognosis; conversely, the remission of psychiatric symptoms correlates with a reduction of physical symptoms.

Inflammatory bowel disease includes ulcerative colitis, other types of colitis, and Crohn's disease. Contrary to earlier findings, recent studies do not demonstrate a bimodal age distribution for inflammatory bowel disease, but rather the prevalence of both Crohn's disease and ulcerative colitis decline after age 40 with only 10% of patients with inflammatory bowel disease being older than 60 years.[46] However, the elderly can be more susceptible to medical complications related to the disease and its treatments.

Peptic ulcer disease can be a result of infection with the bacteria *Helicobacter pylori*. The prevalence of *H pylori* increases with increasing age, making it important to investigate this as a possible cause of anorexia and weight loss in the elderly.[47] Loss of appetite and weight loss are common and can be a result of a number of conditions, including depression or other medical illnesses.

Liver disease is another important gastrointestinal disorder. The hepatitis C virus (HCV) is a common infectious disease that attacks the liver. In most people, HCV tends to be silent and chronic, and usually diagnosed years after the virus was contracted. More than 5 million people in the United States are infected with HCV, and worldwide, the number of people infected reaches 170 million.[48] HCV infection provides an excellent example of the 2-way street between medical and psychiatric illness. Approximately 50% of patients with hepatitis C suffer from a psychiatric illness and are at increased risk for depression.[49] On the one hand, infection with HCV can contribute to depression via multiple mechanisms. Psychologically, it may be depressing to learn that you are infected with the virus and therefore are at risk for complications from HCV, including hepatic insufficiency, cirrhosis, or hepatic failure. It is typical for patients who learn they are infected with HCV to worry that they may have inadvertently infected someone else, including their children or other family members, leading to depressed and anxious mood. Furthermore, there is increasing evidence that HCV may directly cause brain changes and may cross the blood-brain barrier, suggesting that the virus may directly contribute to depressed states.

Conversely, depression can lead to substance abuse, which can result in HCV infection. Currently, sharing needles during intravenous drug use is the most common route for contracting the virus. The severity of the liver damage can be quite variable among individuals with HCV, with some individuals having no evidence of liver impairment and others with serious liver disease or cirrhosis. The severity of liver disease is an important factor in the management of depression in this population. In addition to the usual metabolic changes that occur with aging, metabolic alterations are also associated with liver disease, further compounding this problem for the elderly patient.

Mr C is a 65-year-old White male who was referred by his gastroenterologist for psychiatric evaluation and treatment of suspected depression. He was diagnosed with HCV 4 months ago after his PCP discovered elevated alanine aminotransaminase, aspartate aminotransaminase, and bilirubin levels on routine blood work. Mr C had used intravenous heroin 30 years ago for a 2-year duration during which he shared needles; his suspected route of infection. He experimented with miscellaneous other drugs during this period as well, but for the past 18 years had used only alcohol. His alcohol use had been heavy and steady, drinking an average of a 6-pack of beer per day, but Mr C discontinued his alcohol use 4 months ago, once he learned of his liver impairment. Psychiatric interview revealed that he had never been treated for a psychiatric condition, but endorsed periods of chronic low-grade depression throughout most of his adult life. Since learning of his liver disease, his depression has worsened. He now endorses anhedonia, insomnia, anorexia, difficulty concentrating, a lack of energy, and anxiety, which have been present for at least the past month. Laboratory evaluation revealed elevated liver function tests, all roughly twice the normal limits; however, on physical examination, the patient had no evidence of ascites or hepatic encephalopathy.

Treatment considerations for depression in patients with comorbid gastrointestinal disease include attention to gastrointestinal motility, absorption, and tolerability, especially regarding common antidepressant side effects, such as nausea and vomiting. When selecting an appropriate antidepressant for a patient with liver impairment, consideration should be given to pharmacokinetic processes (absorption, distribution, metabolism, and elimination). Many antidepressants use the cytochrome P450 system. Liver disease can impair metabolism, resulting in potentially toxic levels of antidepressants, particularly important for TCAs. In patients with portal hypertension, blood is shunted around the liver, reducing first-pass metabolism and potentially leading to increased serum levels of oral medications. Patients with hepatic impairment may also suffer from hepatic encephalopathy or delirium due to hepatic insufficiency, which can be further exacerbated by certain drugs, especially those with anticholinergic properties. Ascites can increase the volume of distribution of drugs and decrease serum levels of antidepressants. Dosage adjustments of medications are often necessary to balance the pharmacokinetic effects of hepatic impairment.

All antidepressants currently available in the United States are hepatically metabolized, and elevated plasma concentrations have been demonstrated in patients with hepatic impairment for nearly all of them. Furthermore, clinicians should be aware of the potential for hepatotoxic effects of some antidepressants. There are case reports of hepatic dysfunction associated with the use of TCAs[50] and SSRIs.[51,52] TCAs can cause sedation due to antihistaminic activity and may exacerbate hepatic encephalopathy. When used, they may be used in lower doses and serum levels can be checked.

SUMMARY

The 2-way relationship between depression and medical illness in late life is complex. Although the association between depression and medical illness is apparent, the cause-and-effect relationship remains ill defined. Daily challenges facing clinicians include making an accurate diagnosis and prescribing safe and effective treatment for elderly patients with such comorbidities. Careful consideration should be given to possible confounding factors, such as adverse effects of prescribed medications, alcohol, or other substance use and other physical and environmental factors that may play a role in the patient's outcome.

REFERENCES

1. Nemeroff CB, Owens MJ. The role of serotonin in the pathophysiology of depression: as important as ever. Clin Chem 2009;55:1257S–9.

2. Glassman AH, Shapiro PA. Depression and the course of coronary artery disease. Am J Psychiatry 1998;155(1):4–11.
3. Evans DL, Charney DS, Lewis L, et al. Mood disorders in the medically ill: scientific review and recommendations. Biol Psychiatry 2005;58:175–89.
4. Mallik S, Krumholz HM, Lin ZQ, et al. Patients with depressive symptoms have lower health status benefits after coronary artery bypass surgery. Circulation 2005;111:271–7.
5. Lesperance F, Frasure-Smith N, Talajic M. Major depression before and after myocardial infarction: its nature and consequences. Psychosom Med 1996; 58:99–110.
6. Glassman AH, Bigger JT, Gaffney M. Psychiatric characteristics associated with long-term mortality among 361 patients having an acute coronary syndrome and major depression: seven-year follow-up of SADHART participants. Arch Gen Psychiatry 2009;66(9):1022–9.
7. Glassman AH, O'Connor CM, Califf RM, et al. Sertraline treatment of major depression in patients with acute MI or unstable angina. JAMA 2002;288(6):701–9.
8. Schulz R, Beach SR, Ives DG, et al. Association between depression and mortality in older adults: the cardiovascular health study. Arch Intern Med 2000; 160(12):1761–8.
9. Tiemeier H, van Dijck W, Hofman A, et al. Relationship between atherosclerosis and late-life depression: the Rotterdam study. Arch Gen Psychiatry 2004;61: 369–76.
10. Blazer DG. Depression in late life: review and commentary. J Gerontol A Biol Sci Med Sci 2003;58A(3):249–65.
11. Sheline YI, Pieper CF, Barch DM, et al. Support for the vascular depression hypothesis in late-life depression: results of a 2-site, prospective, antidepressant treatment trial. Arch Gen Psychiatry 2010;67(3):277–85.
12. Kales HC, Maixner DF, Mellow AM. Cerebrovascular disease and late-life depression. Am J Geriatr Psychiatry 2005;13(2):88–98.
13. Rumsfeld JS, Ho PM. Depression and cardiovascular disease: a call for recognition. Circulation 2005;111:250–3.
14. Lichtman JH, Bigger JT, Blumenthal JA, et al. Depression and coronary heart disease: recommendations for screening, referral, and treatment. Circulation 2008;118:1768–75.
15. Stefanatou A, Kouris N, Lekakis J. Treatment of depression in elderly patients with cardiovascular disease: research data and future prospects. Hellenic J Cardiol 2010;51:142–52.
16. Chin SH, Balon R. Depression and cardiovascular disease: a case presentation of depression after the onset of acute coronary event. Prim Psychiatr 2004; 11(2):23, 28.
17. Schindler AE. Thyroid function and postmenopause. Gynecol Endocrinol 2003; 17:79.
18. Harman SM, Metter EJ, Tobin JD, et al. Longitudinal effects of aging on serum total and free testosterone levels in healthy men. Baltimore Longitudinal Study of Aging. J Clin Endocrinol Metab 2001;86:724.
19. Christo PJ. Opioid effectiveness and side effects in chronic pain [review]. Anesthesiol Clin North America 2003;21:699–713.
20. Harris JD. Management of expected and unexpected opioid-related side effects. Clin J Pain 2008;24(Suppl 10):S8–13.
21. Brown R, Balousek S, Mundt M, et al. Methadone maintenance and male sexual dysfunction. J Addict Dis 2005;24:91–106.

22. Daniell HW. Opioid-induced androgen deficiency discussion in opioid contracts. Am J Med 2006;120(9):e21.
23. Swaab DF, Boa AM, Lucassen PJ. The stress system in the human brain in depression and neurodegeneration. Ageing Res Rev 2005;4(2):141–94.
24. Mannino D, Homa D, Akinbami L, et al. Chronic obstructive pulmonary disease surveillance—United States. 1971-2000. MMWR Surveill Summ 2002;51(6):1–16.
25. Maurer J, Rebbapragada V, Borson S, et al. Anxiety and depression in COPD: current understanding, unanswered questions, and research needs. Chest 2008;134:43S–56S.
26. Lacasse Y, Rousseau L, Maltais F. Prevalence of depressive symptoms and depression in patients with severe oxygen dependent chronic obstructive pulmonary disease. J Cardiopulm Rehabil 2001;21:80–6.
27. Ewig S, Torres A. Severe community-acquired pneumonia. Clin Chest Med 1999;20:575–87.
28. Gilman S, Abraham H. A longitudinal study on the order of onset of alcohol dependence and major depression. Drug Alcohol Depend 2005;63(3):277–86.
29. Tashkin D, Kanner R, Bailey W, et al. Smoking cessation in patients with chronic obstructive pulmonary disease: a double-blind, placebo-controlled, randomized trial. Lancet 2001;357:1571–5.
30. Covey L, Glassman A, Stetner F. Depression and depressive symptoms in smoking cessation. Compr Psychiatry 1990;31:350–4.
31. Kenna H, Poon A, de los Angeles P, et al. Psychiatric complications of treatment with corticosteroids: review with case report. Psychiatry Clin Neurosci 2011;65: 549–60.
32. Douglas N. Chronic obstructive pulmonary disease. In: Kruger M, Roth T, Dement W, editors. Principles and practice of sleep medicine. 3rd edition. Philadelphia: WB Saunders; 2000. p. 965–75.
33. Garvey C. Depression in patients with chronic obstructive pulmonary disease. Postgrad Med 2012;124(3):101–9.
34. Hedayati S, Minhajuddin A, Toto R, et al. Prevalence of major depressive episode in CKD. Am J Kidney Dis 2009;54(3):424–32.
35. Hedayati S, Bosworth H, Briley L, et al. Death or hospitalization of patients on chronic hemodialysis is associated with a physician-based diagnosed of depression. Kidney Int 2008;74:930–6.
36. Neu S, Kjellstrand C. Stopping long-term dialysis. N Engl J Med 1986;314: 14–20.
37. Levy N. Psychiatric considerations in the primary medical care of the patient with renal failure. Adv Ren Replace Ther 2000;7(3):231–8.
38. Kalender D, Ozdemir A, Koroglu G. Association of depression with markers of nutrition and inflammation in chronic kidney disease and end-stage renal disease. Nephron Clin Pract 2006;102:115–21.
39. Brown T, Brown R. Neuropsychiatric consequences of renal failure. Psychosomatics 1995;36:244–53.
40. DiMatteo M, Lepper H, Croghan T. Depression is a risk factor for noncompliance with medical treatment meta-analysis of the effects of anxiety and depression of patient adherence. Arch Intern Med 2000;160:2101–7.
41. Loghman-Adham M. Medication noncompliance in patients with chronic disease: issues in dialysis and renal transplantation. Am J Manag Care 2003;9: 155–71.
42. Kimmel P, Cukor D, Cohen S, et al. Depression in end-stage renal disease patients: a critical review. Adv Chronic Kidney Dis 2007;14(4):328–34.

43. Greenwald DA. Aging, the gastrointestinal tract, and the risk of acid-related disease. Am J Med 2004;117(Suppl 5A):8S–13S.
44. Drossman DA. AGA technical review on irritable bowel syndrome. Gastroenterology 2002;123(6):2108.
45. Guthrie EA, Creed F, Whorwell PJ, et al. Outpatients with irritable bowel syndrome: a comparison of first time and chronic attenders. Gut 1992;33:361–3.
46. Cangemi JR. Intestinal ischemia in the elderly. Gastroenterol Clin North Am 2009;38(3):527–40.
47. Salles N. *Helicobacter pylori* infection in elderly patients. Rev Med Interne 2007; 28(6):400–11.
48. Chak E, Talal AH, Sherman KE, et al. Hepatitis C virus infection in USA: an estimate of true prevalence. Liver Int 2011;31(8):1090–101.
49. Yovtcheva SP, Rifai MA, Moles JK, et al. Psychiatric comorbidity among hepatitis C–positive patients. Psychosomatics 2011;42(5):411–5.
50. Pedersen AM, Enevoldsen HK. Nortriptyline-induced hepatic failure. Ther Drug Monit 1996;18:100–2.
51. Cai Q, Benson MA, Talbot TJ, et al. Acute hepatitis due to fluoxetine therapy. Mayo Clin Proc 1999;92:1225–6.
52. De Man RA. Severe hepatitis attributed to paroxetine. Ned Tijdschr Geneeskd 1997;141:540–2.

Assessment of the Person with Late-life Depression

Juliet Glover, MD[a], Shilpa Srinivasan, MD[b],*

KEYWORDS

- Depression • Geriatric depression • Late-life depression • Depression assessment
- Clinical presentation of depression • Clinical evaluation of depression

KEY POINTS

- Thorough assessment for depression in elderly patients includes comprehensive psychiatric interview of the patient and collateral sources.
- Identification of risk factors for late-life depression, suicide risk assessment, functional status evaluation, and assessment of cognitive status are integral to the clinical evaluation and management.
- Laboratory studies and neuroimaging can facilitate identification of associated comorbidities as contributors to the medical or neurologic causes of depression symptoms.
- Validated rating scales can aid in the identification and monitoring of symptoms over time.

INTRODUCTION

Depression in elderly adults is a serious condition with distinct morphologic and clinical features, with first onset after age 65 years. According to the *Diagnostic and Statistical Manual of Mental Disorders, Fourth Edition, Text Revision* (DSM-IV-TR), a major depressive episode is defined as the presence of low mood or anhedonia plus 4 or more associated symptoms occurring nearly all day, daily for 2 or more weeks (**Box 1**).[1] The lifetime prevalence of MDD in the general adult population is estimated at 15% to 17%,[2] whereas the 1-year prevalence rate in individuals ages 65 years and older is lower at 1% to 4%.[3–6] Prevalence rates of MDD are higher in women than in men (4.4% vs 2.7% respectively).[7] Despite the lower prevalence of MDD in the older adult population, an estimated 15% to 25% of older adults suffer from subthreshold symptoms of depression identified by fewer than 5 DSM-IV-TR

[a] Geriatric Psychiatry Fellowship Program, Palmetto Health, University of South Carolina School of Medicine, 3555 Harden Street, Suite 301, Columbia, SC 29203, USA; [b] Department of Neuropsychiatry and Behavioral Sciences, University of South Carolina School of Medicine, 3555 Harden Street, Suite 301, Columbia, SC 29203, USA
* Corresponding author.
E-mail address: Shilpa.srinivasan@uscmed.sc.edu

Psychiatr Clin N Am 36 (2013) 545–560
http://dx.doi.org/10.1016/j.psc.2013.08.004
0193-953X/13/$ – see front matter Published by Elsevier Inc.

Abbreviations: Assessment of Late-life Depression	
AIDS	Acquired Immunodeficiency Syndrome
ADLs	Activities of Daily Living
BDI	Beck Depression Inventory
CDT	Clock Drawing test
CMP	Complete Metabolic Panel
GDS	Geriatric Depression Scale
HAM-D	Hamilton Rating Scale for Depression
HIV	Human Immunodeficiency Virus
IADLs	Instrumental activities of daily living
LLD	Late-life depression
MDD	Major depressive disorder
MMSE	Mini Mental Status Examination
PHQ-9	Patient Health Questionnaire-9
PRIME-MD	Primary Care Evaluation of Mental Disorders
RPR	Rapid plasma reagin
SLUMS	St. Louis University Mental Status exam
T_3	Triiodothyronine
T_4	Thyroxine
TBG	Thyroxine-binding globulin
TSH	Thyroid-stimulating hormone
VDRL	Venereal Disease Research Laboratory

criteria for a major depressive episode being met or, when 5 or more criteria are met, symptoms last less than 2 weeks. These symptoms nevertheless cause distress and functional impairment but do not meet criteria for a major depressive episode or MDD and are classified as minor or subsyndromal depression.[8] The prevalence of both MDD and clinically significant minor depression varies by clinical setting, with the lowest rates observed in community settings and the highest rates in long-term

---

Box 1
DSM-IV-TR criteria for major depressive episode

Five or more of the following symptoms present during the same 2-week period

At least 1 symptom is depressed mood or anhedonia

1. Depressed mood

2. Anhedonia

3. Change in appetite or significant weight loss or weight gain

4. Insomnia or hypersomnia

5. Psychomotor agitation or retardation

6. Fatigue or loss of energy

7. Feelings of worthlessness of excessive or inappropriate guilt

8. Diminished ability to think or concentrate or indecisiveness

9. Recurrent thoughts of death or suicidal ideation

Data from Diagnostic and statistical manual of mental disorders, fourth edition, text revision. Washington, DC: American Psychiatric Association; 2000. http://dx.doi.org/10.1176/appi.books. 9780890423349.

care facilities, where up to 40% of patients exhibit depressive symptoms (**Fig. 1**).[5,9] The growth of the older adult population coupled with prevalence rates of depression underscores the importance of timely recognition and accurate assessment of LLD in this demographic.

According to the World Health Organization 2004 report, depression is the third leading cause of global burden of disease.[10] The impact of LLD is significant and far-reaching. LLD is associated with functional impairment, cognitive decline, increased risk of morbidity and mortality from medical illnesses, along with higher rate of health care use and costs.[3,6,8,11] The impact of medical morbidity and depression seems to be bidirectional. Depression is associated with poor outcomes with comorbid medical illness which, in turn, negatively affects the course of depression.[8,12] In addition to medical morbidity and mortality, suicide mortality is an important consideration in LLD. Older adults are at disproportionately high risk for suicide, with the highest rates in older white men. In 2007, the United States suicide rate for individuals aged 65 to 74 years was 14.3 per 100,000, higher than the national average of 11.3 suicides per 100,000 individuals in the general population. The rate of suicide in non-Hispanic white men aged 85 years or older is even higher at 47 per 100,000.[13]

Individuals born between 1946 and 1964, the so-called baby boomers, are at a higher risk for suicide than earlier and later generations.[14] As this cohort continues to age, it is estimated that suicide rates will increase, further highlighting the importance of adequate assessment and treatment of depression in this patient population.

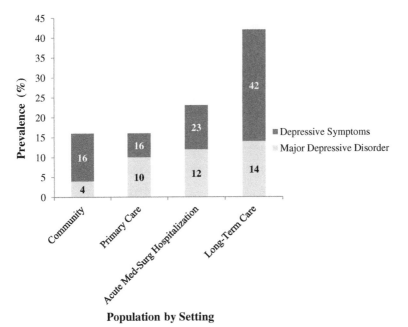

Population by Setting

Fig. 1. Prevalence of late-life depression by health/independence status. (*Data from* Blazer DG. Depression in late life: review and commentary. J Gerontol A Biol Sci Med Sci 2003;58(3):249–65; and Djernes JK. Prevalence and predictors of depression in populations of elderly: a review. Acta Psychiatr Scand 2006;113(5):372–87.)

CLINICAL PRESENTATION OF LLD

Although the diagnostic criteria for major depression are applicable to both general and older adults (see **Box 1**), there are characteristic differences in the clinical presentation of depression in the older adult (**Table 1**). Older adults are more likely to show anhedonia, irritability, or social withdrawal as the presenting symptom of depression.[3] Somatic complaints and neurovegetative changes such as fatigue, changes in appetite, sleep disturbance, poor concentration, and psychomotor retardation are often prominent.[3,15–17] A 2012 meta-analysis by Hegeman and colleagues[17] comparing 11 studies (n = 2000) found that older adults with depression are more likely to present with agitation, somatic complaints (especially gastrointestinal symptoms), and hypochondriasis and less likely to show guilt or loss of sexual interest compared with younger adults. Individuals with LLD are less likely to have a family history of depression or other mental illness than those with early onset symptoms.[5,15] LLD is frequently associated with medical comorbidities, especially cardiovascular disease, whereas early onset depression is often associated with psychosocial comorbidities such as relational discord and personality dysfunction.[18] Recognition of these differences may aid practitioners in accurately identifying depression in the older adult.

IDENTIFICATION OF RISK AND PROTECTIVE FACTORS IN DEPRESSION

When evaluating an older adult, clinicians must be cognizant of factors that increase the risk for depression. These risk factors can be subdivided into biological and psychosocial components. Biological factors that increase the risk for depression include female gender, comorbid substance abuse, chronic pain, sleep disturbance, medical illness, and iatrogenic causes in the form of depressogenic medications. Medical illnesses associated with LLD include cardiovascular disease, stroke, thyroid dysfunction, hip fractures, malignancies, and dementing illnesses to include Alzheimer disease and Parkinson disease. Narcotic pain medications, benzodiazepines, interferon-alfa, antineoplastic agents, and antihypertensives including β-blockers and calcium channel blockers have been linked to depression in older adults.[5,6,15,19] Individuals with prior history of depression or suicide attempt are at increased risk.[3] Psychosocial risk factors include social isolation; single, divorced, or widowed status; individuals with disabilities; poor perceived health status; lower socioeconomic status;

Table 1 Clinical presentation of depression in elderly versus young adults		
Symptom	**Adult Presentation**	**Geriatric Presentation**
Mood	Depressed Anhedonic (reduced interest) Suicidal thoughts	Fatigue, hopelessness Anger, anxiety, irritability Thoughts of death
Somatic	+/− Sleep +/− Appetite +/− Psychomotor +/− Pain	↑ Pain Somatic symptoms overlap with comorbid disease, medications
Cognitive	Reduced concentration Indecisiveness	Reduced selective attention Reduced working memory/retrieval Reduced new learning Reduced processing speed Executive dysfunction

Data from Refs.[3,16–19]

and negative life events, including bereavement and financial difficulties.[3,6,19] Those who serve in the caregiver role are also at increased risk, with depression reported in 25% to 50% of these individuals.[3] Across all categories of risk factors, a 2003 meta-analysis of 20 studies and more than 23,000 subjects found the following 5 risk factors to be significant[6]:

- Bereavement
- Sleep disturbance
- Disability
- Prior depression
- Female gender

Careful attention to these potential indicators of depression may increase identification and foster an in-depth assessment of the patient.

In contrast, certain factors serve as buffers against the development of depression symptoms in older adults, even in the face of adverse life events. One such protective factor is healthy physical and cognitive functioning. Social connectedness and participation in meaningful social activities has also been shown to decrease the risk of depression.[19]

CLINICAL VIGNETTE: OLDER ADULT WITH LLD

S.P. is a 74-year-old retired schoolteacher with no previous history of psychiatric illness. She is referred by her primary care physician because of anergy, fatigue, and anhedonia, as well as complaints of memory loss. Her adult son and daughter accompany her to the visit. S.P. reports that although she loves her children, they get on her nerves and she does not like to do the things they want her to do. She complains of feeling fatigued and attributes it to pain in her back and knees. She is able to fall asleep without difficulty but awakens at 4 AM and is unable to go back to sleep. On further questioning, she admits, "I don't enjoy anything." She also complains of difficulty concentrating and keeping track of events, and of feeling tired all the time. She asks, "Do I have that 'old-timer's disease'?" She gives permission for her children to provide input.

S.P.'s adult children report that their mother has been disinterested, withdrawn, and no longer wants to spend time even with her grandchildren. She no longer cooks, complaining of fatigue, and has been losing weight. They are concerned because S.P. wants to stay in bed for much of the day. They also note that she has been forgetful and requires reminders for birthdays and other events that she normally would not have trouble remembering. Family notes symptom onset 8 months ago, when she moved from out of state after her second husband's death. S.P. had been an avid gardener, and her family notes that she stopped 3 months ago, despite their encouragement.

S.P.'s medical history is significant for hypertension and coronary artery disease with a history of myocardial infarction 5 years ago, type 2 diabetes mellitus, vitamin D deficiency, and osteoarthritis. Her current medications include metoprolol, lisinopril, aspirin, metformin, hydrocodone-acetaminophen, and vitamin D. She also takes sertraline 100 mg daily and alprazolam 0.5 mg twice a day, which she states is for, "not sleeping well since my husband died." There is no history of substance use and family history is negative for mood disorders or other psychiatric illness. S.P. had a normal annual comprehensive physical examination and diagnostic work-up 1 month ago and her medication regimen has been stable for the last 3 months.

On examination, S.P. appears disheveled. Her clothing is clean but frayed. She describes her mood as, "Alright." Her affect is blunted and she becomes tearful when discussing her late husband. She denies suicidal or homicidal ideation. There is no evidence of psychosis. S.P. is alert and oriented to person, place, month, and year. She scores 24/30 on the SLUMS examination. She refuses to complete the clock drawing.

CLINICAL ASSESSMENT OF LLD: THE PSYCHIATRIC INTERVIEW

At the initial visit, the patient should first be interviewed individually to establish rapport, capture a preliminary history, and allow for the assessment of sensitive topics such as suicidal ideation, sexual dysfunction, family conflict, or abuse history. When interviewing the patient, the clinician must be cognizant of sensory impairment, including hearing and visual difficulties, and tailor the interview appropriately to accommodate these impairments while still gathering detailed information and history.

Subsequently obtaining historical information from collateral sources, with the patient's permission, is valuable to the overall assessment. Informants may include the spouse, adult children and other relatives, or caregivers. Family members may be able to provide additional history of symptom onset and course, past psychiatric illness, and premorbid functioning. This additional history is particularly valuable in situations in which the patient lacks insight, denies the presence of a depressive illness, or has cognitive difficulties. Collateral sources may also be able to provide a comprehensive picture of the patient's functional capability because family members may be involved in the daily care of the patient in the home setting.[20]

The components of the psychiatric interview of the older adult are similar to that of younger patient. They include gathering history of present illness, past psychiatric history, medical history, current medications and allergies, family history, social history, and performing a mental status examination. In addition, an assessment of functional status is also crucial to the psychiatric evaluation of an older adult.[20,21]

History of Present Illness

When obtaining the history of present illness, an open-ended approach allows patients to describe their understanding of and explanation for symptoms, which can be followed by more specific and symptom-focused questions. The initial evaluation should include exploration of recent stressors including changes in home environments, recent losses or deaths, financial stress, loss of social support networks, or physical illness that may have precipitated or contributed to onset of symptoms.[20] Any present or past alcohol or substance use, including abuse of prescription medications, should be comprehensively explored.

Past Psychiatric History

Past psychiatric history captured should include ascertaining previous history of similar symptoms/episodes and prior response to treatment modalities.

Medical History, Current Medications, and Family History

The patient's medical history and current medications should be reviewed. The presence of family history of mood or cognitive impairment should be noted. Parents and siblings of older adults may be deceased and age, cause of death, and functional status at time of death should be identified.

Social History

Important elements of the social history include identification of education and work history; marital status; intimate relationships, including an evaluation of sexual activity/functioning; living arrangements; social support networks; and religious affiliations. The social history should not be overlooked because a breakdown in one of the areas discussed earlier may represent the precipitating stressor that leads to onset of depression symptoms.

Functional Status Assessment

A functional status assessment is an integral component of the evaluation, allowing determination of the patients' strengths and weaknesses pertinent to the ability to care for themselves and live independently. The patient's ability to independently complete ADLs (eg, bathing, dressing, grooming, toileting, feeding, and self-transferring) should be identified. IADLs, including ability to drive, shop for groceries, prepare food, manage finances, use the telephone, and safely administer medications, should be evaluated at this stage.[20,22] In a study by Alexopoulos and colleagues,[23] impairment in IADLs was correlated with increased depression severity, anxiety, psychomotor retardation, and weight loss. Severity of depression symptoms and associated cognitive impairment is a predictor of impairment in IADLs.[24] Identification of functional deficits facilitates timely implementation of appropriate interventions into the treatment plan and provides an index of disease severity to be monitored over the course of treatment.[20]

DIFFERENTIAL DIAGNOSIS OF LLD

Differential diagnoses include bipolar spectrum disorders, dysthymia, mood disorder caused by general medical condition, substance-induced or medication-induced mood disorder, depressive disorder not otherwise specified, adjustment disorder with depressed mood, and bereavement.[24,25] The diagnostic criteria for each of these diagnoses are detailed in DSM-IV-TR.[1]

Clinical Assessment of LLD: Mental Status Examination

Key components of the formal mental status examination include:

1. Sensorium and orientation
2. General appearance and behavior
3. Mood and affect
4. Speech
5. Thought process
6. Thought content
7. Perception
8. Cognitive assessment
9. Assessment of insight and judgment

Psychomotor abnormalities may include psychomotor agitation as shown by restlessness or psychomotor retardation related to fatigue, amotivation, and apathy. Delusional content in the older depressed patient may be mood congruent and include delusions of guilt, sin, or hypochondriasis.[20] Disturbances in perception may be in the form of hallucinations, especially auditory or visual hallucinations. A thorough assessment of thought content includes exploration of thoughts of self-harm and suicidal and homicidal ideations or plans.

Screening and Assessment for Suicide

As part of the clinical evaluation, it is essential to screen for suicidal ideation, which can range from passive (thoughts of hopelessness or that life is not worth living), in the absence of intent to self-harm, to active thoughts of self-harm or suicidal ideation. It is necessary to query and explore whether the patient has plans for suicide. Access to weapons or other lethal means such as hoarding of medications should always be ascertained as part of the assessment. Firearms are the most frequently used method of completed suicide in older adults (28%), followed by hanging (24%) and poisoning (21%).[26]

The assessment of suicide includes exploration of risk factors and warning signs. History of previous suicide attempts and presence of a mood disorder are risk factors for suicide. MDD has been associated with greater than 50% of completed suicides.[14] Other suicide risk factors include chronic medical and neurologic illnesses such as HIV/AIDS, chronic obstructive pulmonary disease, congestive heart failure, renal disease, malignancies, chronic pain, Huntington disease, Parkinson disease, multiple sclerosis, seizure disorder, and spinal cord injury.[26,27] Functional impairment in IADLs, often as a result of medical and psychiatric illness, confers heightened risk, particularly when correlated with feelings of guilt and burden.[27,28] Psychosocial factors including rigid or neurotic personality traits, social isolation, family discord, and impending placement in a long-term care facility have also been shown to increase the risk of suicide.[19,27] Suicide risk factors may or may not be modifiable by clinical interventions. In contrast, protective factors serving as buffers against suicide risk in the elderly include spiritual and religious beliefs, cultural attitudes that object to suicide, and overall positive societal attitudes toward older adults.[14,27]

Suicide warning signs are indicators of imminent risk of suicide and should prompt immediate action.[29] Unlike suicide risk factors, which are often static, warning signs can be variable and should be assessed frequently and on an ongoing basis. These signs include thoughts, feelings, and behaviors that indicate preparation for suicide. Warning signs can be summarized with the mnemonic IS PATH WARM (**Box 2**).[29,30] Evaluation of suicide risk and warning signs is critical. However, studies show that clinicians often miss opportunities for intervention. Luoma and colleagues[31] found that 58% of individuals aged 55 years and older had contact with their primary care providers within 1 month of completed suicide, whereas 77% had contact within 1 year of completed suicide. This study also found that 11% of individuals aged 55 years and older had contact with a mental health professional within 1 month and 8.5% within 1 year of completed suicide. These figures underscore the need for thorough assessment of suicide risk and warning signs to facilitate prompt intervention.

Box 2
Suicide warning signs: IS PATH WARM mnemonic

Ideation: talking about death; threatening or looking for ways to hurt self

Substance abuse: increased alcohol or drug use

Purposelessness: no reason to live; feeling no sense of purpose

Anxiety: anxious, agitated, sleep disturbance

Trapped: feeling trapped, like there's no way out

Hopelessness: loss of hope that situation will improve

Withdrawal: withdrawal from family, friends, society

Anger: anger, rage, seeking revenge

Recklessness: engaging in risky behavior

Mood changes: dramatic changes in mood

Date from Rudd MD, Berman AL, Joiner TE Jr, et al. Warning signs for suicide: theory, research, and clinical applications. Suicide Life Threat Behav 2006;36(3):255–62; and The origin of the evidenced-based consensus-developed IS PATH WARM? Warning signs [cited 2012 November]. Available at: http://www.suicidology.org/c/document_library/get_file?folderId=231&name=DLFE-599.pdf. Accessed November 9, 2012.

PHYSICAL EXAMINATION AND LABORATORY STUDIES

Although the clinical interview is paramount in the evaluation and diagnosis of LLD, a thorough physical examination with vigilance for any signs of underlying medical and/or neurologic dysfunction is an essential part of the work-up. Routine laboratory studies should include a complete blood count to rule out anemia, which may contribute to anergy and fatigue in patients with suspected LLD. A CMP including renal and liver function tests should be obtained. The CMP may reveal glucose abnormalities causing weakness or fatigue. A baseline sodium level should be obtained because treatment of depression with certain antidepressants has been associated with development of hyponatremia and syndrome of inappropriate antidiuretic hormone secretion. Abnormal calcium and magnesium levels may result in delusions or psychosis and should be ruled out in cases of suspected MDD with psychotic features.[32] Checking thyroid function panel, including TSH, T_4, T_3, and TBG, can identify hypothyroidism, which may produce symptoms that mimic depression including psychomotor retardation, flat affect, cognitive changes, and gastrointestinal symptoms. TSH can be used as an initial screen and, if abnormal, additional tests of thyroid function should be obtained.[25] Tests for nutritional status, including albumin, vitamin B_{12}, and folate, are part of the initial work-up. Vitamin B_{12} and folate abnormalities may contribute to anemia, depression, and cognitive dysfunction.[32] Screening tests for syphilis including RPR or VDRL may reveal untreated infection that can lead to psychosis and cognitive decline. HIV testing should be considered, especially if cognitive impairment is prominent, given that AIDS can lead to cognitive decline. A urine drug screen may reveal comorbid prescription or illicit substance use disorder including benzodiazepine, barbiturate, opioid, and cocaine use, all of which may lead to depression symptoms.[32] Testing 25-hydroxyvitamin D levels should be considered because studies have shown a relationship between low levels of vitamin D and depression.[33–37]

In addition to the aforementioned routine tests, LLD has been associated with other endocrine abnormalities that are not routinely tested, but may be considered. These abnormalities include increased secretion of corticotropin-releasing factor and nonsuppression of cortisol on the dexamethasone suppression test. Decreased levels of sex hormones, including low testosterone, have also been associated with depression symptoms.[5]

DEPRESSION RATING SCALES

Standardized screening tools and rating scales should be used as part of the clinical examination to aid in identification of depression. Such scales can aid in screening and, in some cases, monitoring of response to treatment. However, they do not replace the psychiatric interview. Although there are several rating scales commonly used in clinical practice, 4 commonly used, standardized screening and rating scales validated for use in the geriatric population are discussed in more detail later. These scales include the GDS, PHQ-9, BDI, and HAM-D.

GDS

The GDS is a screening instrument developed specifically for the older adult population.[18,20]

- It can either be self-administered or administered by a clinician and takes approximately 5 to 7 minutes to complete.[3]

- The GDS is particularly useful in the elderly population because of its simple Yes/No format and focus on issues related to cognition, loss, and self-image as opposed to neurovegetative symptoms that may be related to medical illness.[21]
- The presence of 5 or more depression symptom responses suggests a positive screen for depression.[15]
- GDS has shown validity in inpatient and outpatient settings and has overall sensitivity of 84% and specificity of 95%.[3]
- The original instrument consists of 30 questions, although shorter 15-item and ultrashort 4-item and 5-item versions have been developed.
- A 2009 meta-analysis compared sensitivities and specificities of the 30-item, 15-item, and 4-item or 5-item versions in identifying depression in community medical and nursing home settings and found the ultrashort version to have the highest sensitivity, at 92.5%. The specificity of this version was reported at 77.2% and was similar to the longer versions.[11]
- The validity and brevity of this instrument may make it a favorable choice for busy primary care providers.

PHQ-9

The PHQ-9 is a 9-item depression screening tool originally designed for use in primary care settings and derived from the PRIME-MD rating scale.[38] The use of PHQ-9 in nursing homes and community settings has also been shown.[39,40]

- The PHQ-9 consists of 9 items that correspond with the DSM-IV-TR criteria for major depressive episode. Patients are asked to score each item on a scale of 0 to 3, based on frequency of occurrence over the preceding 2-week period. Depression symptoms can then be rated as follows: score of less than 5, no depression; 5 to 9, mild depression; 10 to 14 = moderate depression; 15 to 19, moderately severe depression; and 20 to 27, severe depression.[18,39] When monitoring response to treatment, a decrease of at least 5 points indicates clinically significant improvement.[39]
- Like the GDS, it can either be administered by a clinician or self-administered.
- The PHQ-9 has been shown to be both sensitive and specific (>80%).[40]
- A shorter 2-item version, the PHQ-2, consists of the first 2 items of the PHQ-9, which ask about depressed mood and anhedonia, and has reported sensitivity of 80% and specificity of 78%.[40]
- The PHQ-2 can be used as an initial screening tool and those who screen positive can then be administered the PHQ-9. This 2-step process has been shown to have similar sensitivity and specificity to the PHQ-9 and has the added advantage of saving time by eliminating the administration of the longer PHQ-9 to those who screen negative on the PHQ-2.[40]
- Overall, the advantages of the PHQ are its correspondence with DSM-IV-TR criteria for major depression, ease of administration, validation in older adults and different settings, and usefulness in monitoring response to treatment.

BDI

The BDI is a 21-item self-report rating instrument that is useful for both screening and assessing severity of depression symptoms.[41] Although the BDI has shown validity and reliability when used with older adult populations,[42,43] a 2002 study comparing the responses of older versus younger patients found that older adults tend to report more somatic complaints than cognitive symptoms such as guilt and self-criticism.[41]

A primary care version provides a shorter version of the original BDI that consists of 7 questions and excludes somatic symptoms in order to decrease false-positive rates from comorbid medical problems.[41]

HAM-D

The HAM-D was not designed specifically as a screening tool, but it is most effective for monitoring symptoms and response to treatment.[3,21]

- Like the BDI, the HAM-D is a clinician-administered and clinician-rated tool.
- Given its length and the clinician training that is required to administer it, it is used more often in research than in clinical settings.
- One disadvantage in using this scale in the elderly population with high prevalence of comorbid medical illness is the large number of questions related to somatic symptoms.[20]

COGNITION AND LLD

Cognitive deficits, especially reduced processing speed and executive dysfunction, are associated with depression in the elderly. These deficits may be secondary to depression or may represent an underlying cognitive disorder, such as dementia. Chronology of symptom onset may assist in determining whether cognitive issues are related to depression. In cases in which symptoms of depression precede onset of cognitive changes, depression is more likely to be the cause of the cognitive impairment. In these cases, the cognitive deficit, also termed dementia syndrome of depression, may be reversible with treatment of depression.[3] LLD is associated with increased risk for subsequent development of dementia. LLD may be a risk factor or represent a prodrome of dementia.[44] In contrast, if cognitive decline precedes onset of depression, it is important to consider co-occurring dementia.[19] Major depression has been reported in up to 20% of patients with Alzheimer dementia.[5] Given the association between LLD and cognitive changes, it is important to include cognitive testing in the clinical evaluation of an older adult with depression. Essential aspects of the cognitive assessment as part of the mental status examination include tests of orientation, recent and remote memory, language, fund of knowledge, and attention/concentration.[20,21] Formal cognitive screening tools, including the Folstein MMSE, SLUMS examination, and the Mini-Cog are reviewed in more detail later.

Folstein MMSE

The MMSE is a 19-item, 30-point screening tool for cognitive dysfunction developed in 1975.[45] MMSE scores are affected by age, level of education, and cultural background.

- The test takes approximately 10 minutes to administer and can be administered at different time points to measure longitudinal changes in cognitive status.[46]
- The cutoff scores for the Standardized MMSE, a variation of the original MMSE in which test instructions are standardized, are as follows:
  - 26 to 30 = normal
  - 25 to 20 = mild cognitive impairment
  - 20 to 10 = moderate impairment
  - 0 to 9 = severe impairment
- Elderly depressed patients often perform poorly on the MMSE, although the poor test performance is incongruent with expected level of disability. This finding is

often a result of apathy or poor effort and the presence of this disability gap may suggest depression versus dementia.

SLUMS Examination

The SLUMS is an 11-item, 30-point screening test developed in 2006.

- It is similar to the MMSE but also includes immediate recall of details from a short story and the CDT for executive function.[47]
- SLUMS cutoff scores are calibrated according to highest level of education.
- It has been shown to be both sensitive and specific (sensitivity 0.92% and specificity 0.81% for those with less than high school education, and sensitivity 0.95% and specificity 0.76% for those with at least a high school education).[48]
- Although it is reported to have similar sensitivity and specificity to the MMSE in the detection of dementia, the SLUMS may be better able to detect mild cognitive impairment.[47]

Mini-Cog

The Mini-Cog is a brief 2-step cognitive screening tool consisting of a 3-item registration and recall test followed by the CDT.[49] Zero out of 3 items recalled indicates a positive screen for cognitive impairment. A normal screen (no cognitive impairment) is indicated by all 3 items being recalled.

- Individuals with intermediate scores (1–2 items recalled) then undergo the CDT and, if abnormal, screen positive for cognitive impairment.
- The Mini-Cog has shown good sensitivity and specificity (80% or greater) in detecting cognitive impairment.[50]
- It is less influenced by level of education and cultural background.[51]
- In addition, it takes approximately 3 minutes to administer, making it preferable in primary care settings.[50,51]
- Its usefulness in the depressed older adult without comorbid dementia is uncertain given that it does not distinguish cognitive impairments that may be caused solely by depression from those that are caused by dementia.

VASCULAR DEPRESSION AND THE ROLE OF NEUROIMAGING

Cerebrovascular disease can predispose, precipitate, or perpetuate depression symptoms in susceptible older adults.[52] Vascular depression has been defined as[3]:

1. Onset of depression symptoms after age 65 years with change in symptoms after vascular event
2. The presence of clinical or laboratory evidence of vascular disease or risk factors

Individuals with vascular depression have associated psychomotor changes including apathy and anergy, cognitive impairment with greater likelihood of progression to dementia, lower likelihood of having a family history of depression, and reduced response to antidepressant treatment.[53] Although a direct causal relationship between cerebrovascular disease and LLD has not been established, associations between the two have been observed.[22] Cerebrovascular lesions are thought to disrupt both gray and white matter tracts.[54] In a 2012 meta-analysis by Sexton and colleagues,[55] vascular depression was correlated with gray matter volume loss in the hippocampus, orbitofrontal cortex, thalamus, and putamen. Disruption of white matter tracts in the frontal and temporal lobes has also been described.[54,56] These findings suggest a role for neuroimaging in the assessment of depression in the elderly when vascular depression is suspected. In these cases, magnetic resonance imaging may reveal white matter hyperintensities,[5] although the influence of lesion location or lesion burden on depression symptoms remains unclear.[53]

SUMMARY

As the population continues to age, health care providers are likely to encounter more elderly patients with depressive symptoms and LLD. Thorough assessment includes comprehensive psychiatric interview of the patient and collateral sources. Identification of risk factors for LLD, suicide risk assessment, functional status evaluation, and assessment of cognitive status are integral to the clinical evaluation and management. Laboratory studies and neuroimaging can facilitate identification of associated comorbidities as contributors to the medical or neurologic causes of depression symptoms. Validated rating scales can aid in the identification and monitoring of symptoms over time. A comprehensive approach to patient assessment is critical to ensure timely and accurate identification and treatment of LLD.

REFERENCES

1. Diagnostic and statistical manual of mental disorders, fourth edition, text revision. Washington, DC: American Psychiatric Association; 2000. http://dx.doi.org/10.1176/appi.books.9780890423349. Accessed September 5, 2013.
2. Kessler RC, Berglund P, Demler O, et al. The epidemiology of major depressive disorder: results from the National Comorbidity Survey Replication (NCS-R). JAMA 2003;289(23):3095–105.
3. Ellison JM, Kyomen HH, Harper DG. Depression in later life: an overview with treatment recommendations. Psychiatr Clin North Am 2012;35(1):203–29.
4. Hasin DS, Goodwin RD, Stinson FS, et al. Epidemiology of major depressive disorder: results from the national epidemiologic survey on alcoholism and related conditions. Arch Gen Psychiatry 2005;62(10):1097–106.
5. Blazer DG. Depression in late life: review and commentary. J Gerontol A Biol Sci Med Sci 2003;58(3):249–65.
6. Cole MG, Dendukuri N. Risk factors for depression among elderly community subjects: a systematic review and meta-analysis. Am J Psychiatry 2003; 160(6):1147–56.
7. Steffens DC, Skoog I, Norton MC, et al. Prevalence of depression and its treatment in an elderly population: the Cache County study. Arch Gen Psychiatry 2000;57(6):601–7.
8. McKinney BC, Sibille E. The age-by-disease interaction hypothesis of late-life depression. Am J Geriatr Psychiatry 2012;10:1–15.
9. Djernes JK. Prevalence and predictors of depression in populations of elderly: a review. Acta Psychiatr Scand 2006;113(5):372–87.
10. World Health Organization. Global burden of disease 2004 update [cited 2012 November]. Available at: http://www.who.int/healthinfo/global_burden_disease/2004_report_update/en/index.html. Accessed November 9, 2012.
11. Mitchell AJ, Bird V, Rizzo M, et al. Which version of the geriatric depression scale is most useful in medical settings and nursing homes? Diagnostic validity meta-analysis. Am J Geriatr Psychiatry 2010;18(12):1066–77.
12. Schulz R, Drayer RA, Rollman BL. Depression as a risk factor for non-suicide mortality in the elderly. Biol Psychiatry 2002;52(3):205–25.
13. Centers for Disease Control and Prevention, National Center for Injury Prevention and Control. Web-Based Injury Statistics Query and Reporting System

(Wisqars). Available at: www.Cdc.Gov/Ncipc/Wisqars. Accessed November 9, 2012.

14. Conwell Y, Van Orden K, Caine ED. Suicide in older adults. Psychiatr Clin North Am 2011;34(2):451–68, ix.

15. Wilkins CH, Mathews J, Sheline YI. Late life depression with cognitive impairment: evaluation and treatment. Clin Interv Aging 2009;4:51–7.

16. Lavretsky H, Kumar A. Clinically significant non-major depression: old concepts, new insights. Am J Geriatr Psychiatry 2002;10(3):239–55.

17. Hegeman JM, Kok RM, van der Mast RC, et al. Phenomenology of depression in older compared with younger adults: meta-analysis. Br J Psychiatry 2012; 200(4):275–81.

18. Balsis S, Cully JA. Comparing depression diagnostic symptoms across younger and older adults. Aging Ment Health 2008;12(6):800–6.

19. Fiske A, Wetherell JL, Gatz M. Depression in older adults. Annu Rev Clin Psychol 2009;5:363–89.

20. Silver I, Herrmann N. Comprehensive psychiatric evaluation. In: Sadavoy J, Jarvik L, Grossberg G, et al, editors. Comprehensive textbook of geriatric psychiatry. 3rd edition. New York: WW Norton &Company; 2004. p. 253–80.

21. Blazer DG. The psychiatric interview of older adults. In: Blazer D, Steffens D, Busse E, editors. Textbook of geriatric psychiatry. 3rd edition. Arlington (VA): American Psychiatric Publishing; 2004. p. 165–77.

22. Alexopoulos G. Late-life mood disorders. In: Sadavoy J, Jarvik L, Grossberg G, et al, editors. Comprehensive textbook of geriatric psychiatry. 3rd edition. New York: WW Norton &Company; 2004. p. 609–43.

23. Alexopoulos GS, Vrontou C, Kakuma T, et al. Disability in geriatric depression. Am J Psychiatry 1996;153(7):877–85.

24. Kiosses DN, Alexopoulos GS. IADL functions, cognitive deficits, and severity of depression: a preliminary study. Am J Geriatr Psychiatry 2005;13(3): 244–9.

25. Koenig H, Blazer D. Mood disorders. In: Blazer D, Steffens D, Busse E, editors. Textbook of geriatric psychiatry. 3rd edition. Arlington (VA): American Psychiatric Publishing; 2004. p. 241–68.

26. Juurlink DN, Herrmann N, Szalai JP, et al. Medical illness and the risk of suicide in the elderly. Arch Intern Med 2004;164(11):1179–84.

27. Van Orden K, Conwell Y. Suicides in late life. Curr Psychiatry Rep 2011;13(3): 234–41.

28. Conwell Y, Duberstein PR, Hirsch JK, et al. Health status and suicide in the second half of life. Int J Geriatr Psychiatry 2010;25(4):371–9.

29. Rudd MD, Berman AL, Joiner TE Jr, et al. Warning signs for suicide: theory, research, and clinical applications. Suicide Life Threat Behav 2006;36(3): 255–62.

30. The origin of the evidenced-based consensus-developed IS PATH WARM? Warning signs [cited 2012 November]. Available at: http://www.suicidology. org/c/document_library/get_file?folderId=231&name=DLFE-599.pdf. Accessed November 9, 2012.

31. Luoma JB, Martin CE, Pearson JL. Contact with mental health and primary care providers before suicide: a review of the evidence. Am J Psychiatry 2002; 159(6):909–16.

32. Taylor W, Doraiswamy P. Use of the laboratory in the diagnostic workup of older adults. In: Blazer D, Steffens D, Busse E, editors. Textbook of geriatric

psychiatry. 3rd edition. Arlington (VA): American Psychiatric Publishing; 2004. p. 179–88.

33. Milaneschi Y, Shardell M, Corsi AM, et al. Serum 25-hydroxyvitamin D and depressive symptoms in older women and men. J Clin Endocrinol Metab 2010;95(7):3225–33.

34. Hoogendijk WJ, Lips P, Dik MG, et al. Depression is associated with decreased 25-hydroxyvitamin D and increased parathyroid hormone levels in older adults. Arch Gen Psychiatry 2008;65(5):508–12.

35. Wilkins CH, Sheline YI, Roe CM, et al. Vitamin D deficiency is associated with low mood and worse cognitive performance in older adults. Am J Geriatr Psychiatry 2006;14(12):1032–40.

36. Brouwer-Brolsma EM, Feskens EJ, Steegenga WT, et al. Associations of 25-hydroxyvitamin D with fasting glucose, fasting insulin, dementia and depression in European elderly: the SENECA study. Eur J Nutr 2012;52(3):917–25.

37. Bertone-Johnson ER, Powers SI, Spangler L, et al. Vitamin D supplementation and depression in the Women's Health Initiative calcium and vitamin D trial. Am J Epidemiol 2012;176(1):1–13.

38. Spitzer RL, Kroenke K, Williams JB. Validation and utility of a self-report version of PRIME-MD: the PHQ primary care study. Primary Care Evaluation of Mental Disorders. Patient Health Questionnaire. JAMA 1999;282(18):1737–44.

39. Kroenke K, Spitzer RL, Williams JB, et al. The patient health questionnaire somatic, anxiety, and depressive symptom scales: a systematic review. Gen Hosp Psychiatry 2010;32(4):345–59.

40. Richardson TM, He H, Podgorski C, et al. Screening depression aging services clients. Am J Geriatr Psychiatry 2010;18(12):1116–23.

41. Kim Y, Pilkonis PA, Frank E, et al. Differential functioning of the Beck Depression Inventory in late-life patients: use of item response theory. Psychol Aging 2002; 17(3):379–91.

42. Gallagher D, Breckenridge J, Steinmetz J, et al. The Beck Depression Inventory and research diagnostic criteria: congruence in an older population. J Consult Clin Psychol 1983;51(6):945–6.

43. Gallagher D, Nies G, Thompson LW. Reliability of the Beck Depression Inventory with older adults. J Consult Clin Psychol 1982;50(1):152–3.

44. Barnes DE, Yaffe K, Byers AL, et al. Midlife vs late-life depressive symptoms and risk of dementia: differential effects for Alzheimer disease and vascular dementia. Arch Gen Psychiatry 2012;69(5):493–8.

45. Folstein MF, Folstein SE, McHugh PR. "Mini-mental state". A practical method for grading the cognitive state of patients for the clinician. J Psychiatr Res 1975; 12(3):189–98.

46. Vertesi A, Lever JA, Molloy DM, et al. Standardized mini-mental state examination. Use and interpretation. Can Fam Physician 2001;47:2018–23.

47. Tariq SH, Tumosa N, Chibnall JT, et al. Comparison of the Saint Louis University mental status examination and the mini-mental state examination for detecting dementia and mild neurocognitive disorder–a pilot study. Am J Geriatr Psychiatry 2006;14(11):900–10.

48. Feliciano L, Horning SM, Klebe K, et al. Utility of the SLUMS as a cognitive screening tool among a nonveteran sample of older adults. Am J Geriatr Psychiatry 2012;21(7):623–30.

49. Borson S. The Mini-Cog: a cognitive "vitals signs" measure for dementia screening in multi-lingual elderly. Int J Geriatr Psychiatry 2000;15(11):1021.

50. Brodaty H, Low LF, Gibson L, et al. What is the best dementia screening instrument for general practitioners to use? Am J Geriatr Psychiatry 2006;14(5): 391–400.

51. Ismail Z, Rajji TK, Shulman KI. Brief cognitive screening instruments: an update. Int J Geriatr Psychiatry 2010;25(2):111–20.

52. Alexopoulos GS, Meyers BS, Young RL, et al. 'Vascular depression' hypothesis. Arch Gen Psychiatry 1997;54(10):915–22.

53. Naismith SL, Norrie LM, Mowszowski L, et al. The neurobiology of depression in later-life: clinical, neuropsychological, neuroimaging and pathophysiological features. Prog Neurobiol 2012;98(1):99–143.

54. Sexton CE, Le Masurier M, Allan CL, et al. Magnetic resonance imaging in late-life depression: vascular and glucocorticoid cascade hypotheses. Br J Psychiatry 2012;201(1):46–51.

55. Sexton CE, Mackay CE, Ebmeier KP. A systematic review and meta-analysis of magnetic resonance imaging studies in late-life depression. Am J Geriatr Psychiatry 2012;21(2):184–95.

56. Firbank MJ, Lloyd AJ, Ferrier N, et al. A volumetric study of MRI signal hyperintensities in late-life depression. Am J Geriatr Psychiatry 2004;12(6):606–12.

Psychological Treatment of Late-Life Depression

Jennifer L. Francis, PhD*, Anand Kumar, MD

KEYWORDS

- Late-life depression • Geriatric depression • Psychiatric interventions
- Cognitive behavioral therapy

KEY POINTS

- Psychological interventions are effective for late-life depression.
- There is little evidence that one type of intervention is more efficacious than another.
- More research is needed to examine moderators of treatment, including age, depression severity, medical illness, and cognitive impairment.

INTRODUCTION

Major depressive disorder (MDD) affects up to 5% of community-dwelling individuals age 55 and older[1] and up to 15% have clinically significant depressive symptoms.[2] Prevalence rates for depression are higher in specialty settings, including primary care (5%–10%)[3] and residential care (10%–50%).[4] Evidence-based guidelines for treatment recommend antidepressants and psychotherapy as the first-line treatment for moderate to severe depression in older adults[5] and this appears to somewhat reflect what occurs in clinical practice. An American Psychiatric Association poll[6] reported that 52% of providers used a combination of medication and therapy and 39% reported prescribing medication only. There is some indication that older adults may prefer psychological treatment compared with pharmacologic treatments,[7,8] and a recent meta-analysis reported that psychotherapy may be more beneficial than antidepressants for older adults with dysthymia and minor depression.[9]

This review examines the evidence for the following psychological interventions in the treatment of late-life depression: cognitive and behavioral therapy, problem-solving therapy, reminiscence and life review therapy, brief psychodynamic therapy, and interpersonal therapy. Following the review of psychological interventions for

Disclosures: None.
Department of Psychiatry, University of Illinois at Chicago, 912 South Wood Street (M/C 913), Chicago, IL 60622, USA
* Corresponding author. Department of Psychiatry (MC 913), University of Illinois at Chicago, 912 South Wood Street, Chicago, IL 60622.
E-mail address: jfrancis@psych.uic.edu

Psychiatr Clin N Am 36 (2013) 561–575
http://dx.doi.org/10.1016/j.psc.2013.08.005
0193-953X/13/$ – see front matter © 2013 Elsevier Inc. All rights reserved.

Abbreviations: Psychological Treatment of Late-Life Depression	
Comm	Community
RDC	Research Diagnostic Criteria
MDD	Major depressive disorder
BDI	Beck Depression Inventory
BT	Behavior therapy
CT	Cognitive therapy
BPD	Brief psychodynamic therapy
WLC	Waitlist control
Indiv	Individual
SADS	Schedule for Affective Disorders and Schizophrenia
HRSD	Hamilton rating scale for depression
GDS	Geriatric Depression Scale
BSI	Brief Symptom Inventory
tx	Treatment
biblio	Bibliotherapy
Unk	Unknown
depx	Depression
bsl	Baseline
CBT	Cognitive behavior therapy
Desip	Desipramine
EDS	Edinburgh Depression Scale
CIDI	Composite International Diagnostic Interview
HTN	Hypertension
HLD	Hyperlipidemia
DISH	Depression Interview and Structured Hamilton
HDI	Hamilton Depression Inventory
TAU	Treatment as usual
AGECAT	Automated Geriatric Examination for Computer Assisted Taxonomy
TC	Talking control
IPT	Interpersonal therapy
SCID	Structured clinical interview
inpt	Inpatient
IPC	Interpersonal counseling
PST	Problem solving therapy
RT	Reminiscence therapy
HSCL-D	Hopkins Symptom Checklist Depression Scale
Exec Dys	Executive dysfunction
ST	Supportive therapy
PC	Primary care
CBP	Community-based psychotherapy
DFDs	Depression-free days
Med Ill	Medically ill
SRT	Structured reminiscence therapy
USRT	Unstructured reminiscence therapy
CESD	Center for Epidemiologic Studies for Depression
LRT	Life review therapy
NT	Narrative therapy

late-life depression, a clinical vignette is presented to provide an example of cognitive behavioral therapy in an older adult with late-life depression.

Methods

Studies were selected through literature searches of PubMed and PsychINFO using combinations of the following key words: cognitive behavior therapy, problem-solving therapy, reminiscence, life review, brief psychodynamic therapy, interpersonal therapy AND late life depression, older adults, and elderly. The reference lists of articles, previous meta-analyses, and reviews were also examined. We included studies that used a randomized, clinical trial with adults 55 years or older who endorsed symptomatic levels of depression based on self-report or clinician interview. Subthreshold levels of depression were included. The sample could be recruited from any setting, as long as the presence of elevated depressive symptoms was part of the inclusion criteria. The experimental intervention was required to be compared with a nonactive control (eg, waitlist control), active control (eg, supportive therapy), treatment as usual (TAU), or another established treatment, either psychological or pharmacologic. Studies had to include a sample size of at least 20 participants in each treatment condition and at least one treatment arm with a psychological intervention as a stand-alone treatment. A total of 17 studies met criteria to be included in the review (**Table 1**) and are discussed as follows by type of intervention.

INTERVENTIONS
Cognitive and Behavioral Therapies

Cognitive and behavioral therapies (CBTs) are a group of evidence-based treatments that combine behavioral and cognitive techniques and have demonstrated efficacy for a wide variety of psychiatric problems, including depression.[10] Cognitive therapy developed by Beck[11] is based on the theory that how we interpret situations impacts our mood and behaviors. Treatment is designed to teach individuals to identify maladaptive or distorted cognitions and learn to challenge them so as to reduce intensity of emotion and problematic behaviors. Behavior therapy for depression is based on the theory that depressed individuals engage in few pleasurable and/or mastery activities and thus do not obtain reinforcement from their environment.[12] Treatment involves increasing pleasurable and mastery activities and uses techniques, such as activity monitoring and scheduling.

A number of meta-analyses have reported large effect sizes for CBT compared with controls in the treatment of late-life depression but no difference between CBT and other established psychological treatments.[13–15] Effects of CBT were weaker when compared with active controls[14] and when examining those with MDD only (vs subthreshold depression).[13]

A total of 7 studies with 12 comparison groups met criteria for this review. CBT treatments included bibliotherapy, and individual, group, and Internet formats. CBT demonstrated significant reduction in depressive symptoms compared with waitlist controls.[16,17] The data were inconsistent when CBT was compared with TAU in 2 primary care samples. Laidlaw and colleagues[18] found no difference between individual CBT and TAU, whereas Serfaty and colleagues[19] reported significantly greater reduction in depressive symptoms compared with TAU. There are several possibilities for the discrepancy. Laidlaw and colleagues[18] had a rather small sample size, suggesting there may not have been enough power to demonstrate differences. Additionally, in both studies, the general practitioner provided TAU but was not blinded in the Serfaty and colleagues[19] study. In fact, the general practitioners (GPs) in the study by Serfaty and colleagues[19] were informed of treatment allocation with the explicit goal of attempting to reduce therapy referrals in the TAU group. Thus, it is possible that the GPs in the study by Serfaty and colleagues[19] did not engage in TAU, whereas Laidlaw and colleagues[18] TAU group received actual TAU.

CBT was not more effective than brief psychodynamic therapy,[20,21] desipramine, or combined desipramine plus CBT.[22] Finally, no differences in reduction of depressive

Table 1
Randomized clinical trials for the treatment of late-life depression included in this review

Study	Total n	Setting	Age	Depression Inclusion Criteria	Conditions	n	Format	Outcome Measures	Assessment Times	Results
Thompson et al,[20] 1987	91	Comm	≥60	RDC MDD ≥17 BDI ≥14 HRSD	1. BT 2. CT 3. BPD 4. WLC	25 27 24 19	Indiv	SADS MDD BDI HRSD GSD BSI	Bsl 6 wk Post tx	BT, CT, BPD > WLC No difference among BT, CT, or BPD
Scogin et al,[16] 1989	67	Comm	≥60	≥10 HRSD	1. BT biblio 2. CT biblio 3. WLC	23 22 22	Indiv	HRSD GDS	Bsl Post Tx 6-mo f/u	CT biblio > WLC on HRSD, GDS BT biblio > WLC on HRSD No sig diff between CT and BT biblio Tx gains maintained at 6 mo
Gallagher-Thompson et al,[21] 1994	66	Comm	Unk	RDC dx of major, minor or intermittent depx disorder ≥10 BDI	1. CBT 2. BPD	36 30	Indiv	SADS HRSD BDI GDS	Bsl 10 wk Post-tx 3 mo 12 mo	CBT = BPD in remission rates Interaction effect for HRSD, BDI, GDS: Caregivers with 3.5 y had more improvement with CBT Caregivers with <3.5 y improved more with BPD
Thompson et al,[22] 2001	102	Comm	≥60	RDC MDD by SADS ≥14 HRSD ≥16 BDI	1. CBT 2. Desipramine 3. CBT + Desipramine	31 33 36	Indiv	SADS HRSD BDI	Bsl Post-tx	All groups effective CBT + Desip > desip alone CBT alone = CBT + desip CBT + Desip better for severely depressed group
Strachowski et al,[17] 2008	48	Comm HTN HLD	≥55	MDD DISH >10 BDI	1. CBT 2. WLC	23 25	Indiv	BDI HDI	Bsl Post tx	CBT > WLC

Study	N	Setting	Age	Inclusion	Conditions	n	Format	Measures	Assessment	Results
Laidlaw et al,[18] 2008	40	PC	≥60	MDD SADS 7–24 HDRS 13–28 BDI	1. CBT 2. TAU	20 20	Indiv	SADS HRSD BDI GDS	Bsl Post tx 3 mo 6 mo	CBT = TAU % remission higher for CBT at post tx and 3 mo but no difference at 6 mo
Serfaty et al,[19] 2009	167	PC	≥65	MDD AGECAT ≥5 GDS ≥14 BDI	1. CBT 2. TC 3. TAU	59 56 52	Indiv	BDI	Bsl 4 mo 10 mo	CBT > TC, TAU
van Schaik et al,[30] 2006	129	Med Clinic	≥55	>5 GDS-15 Prime-MD +MDD	1. IPT 2. TAU	55 74	Indiv	PRIME-MD GDS-15 Remission <10 MADRS Response 50% reduction	Bsl 2 mo 6 mo	Both IP and TAU has reductions in GDS; No sig diff in remission or response or severity between IPT and TAU at 2 mo IPT had significantly more participants w/o Prime-MD diagnosis at 6 mo
Mossey et al,[31] 1996	76	Med inpt	≥60	≥11 GDS No MDD dx SCID	1. IPC 2. TAU 3. Nondepressed control	35 41 77	Indiv	GDS	Bsl 3 mo 6 mo	Both TAU and IPC had sig reductions in GDS at 3 mo but no group difference At 6 mo, IPC significantly lower GDS score and percentage of individuals with GDS score <11 stat sig.
Arean et al,[36] 1993	75	Comm	55+ <80	MDD RDC ≥20 BDI ≥10 GDS ≥18 HAM-D	1. PST 2. RT 3. WLC	28 27 20	Group Group Group	BDI HAM-D GDS	Bsl Post tx 3 mo	PST less depx'd than RT by HRSD and GDS but not BDI PST + RT sig reduced at post tx PST + RT lower scores than WLC

(continued on next page)

Table 1
(continued)

Study	Total n	Setting	Age	Depression Inclusion Criteria	Conditions	n	Format	Outcome Measures	Assessment Times	Results
Williams et al,[40] 2000	415	PC	60+	Dysthymia or minor depx DSM-IIR criteria PRIME-MD ≥10 HDRS	1. PST 2. Paxil 10–40 mg 3. Placebo	138 137 140	Indiv	HSCL-D-20 HDRS-17	Bsl 6 wk 11 wk	PST not greater than paxil or placebo
Arean et al,[38] 2010	221	Comm Exec Dys	60+	MDD SCID >20 HAM-D	1. PST 2. ST	110 111	Group	HAM-D	Bsl 3 wk 9 wk 12 wk (post-tx)	Reductions in PST and ST; PST > improvement at 12 wk vs ST PST > remission and response rates vs ST at 12 wk
Arean et al,[39] 2008	433	PC	60+	MDD or dysthymia by SCID	1. PST-PC 2. PST-PC only 3. CBP 4. CBP only	269 85 164 46	Indiv	HSCL-D-20 DFDs	Bsl 6 mo 12 mo 24 mo	PST-PC only had more DFDs at 12 and 24 mo vs CBP PST-PC lower HSCL-D scores vs CBP at 12 mo but not 24 mo PST-PC with meds still greater than CBP w/meds

Study	N	Setting	Age	Diagnosis	Intervention	N	Format	Measure	Timepoints	Results
Gellis et al,[37] 2008	62	Home Med III	65+	Minor depression by PRIME-MD >10 HRSD	1. PST 2. TAU	30 32	Indiv	HRSD GDS-15	Pre Post 3 mo 6 mo	PST better than TAU
Fry,[50] 1983	162	Comm	65+	>19 BDI	SRT URT Attention control	54 54 54	Indiv	BDI	Bsl Post-tx 15 wk post-tx	SRT < URT SRT, URT < No tx
Serrano et al,[48] 2004	43	Psych Social service	65+	≥16 CESD	Life review TAU (social services)	20 23	Indiv	CESD CIDI	Bsl Post tx	Life review better than TAU Less dx of MDD in life review group vs control at post-tx
Korte et al,[49] 2012	202	Comm	55+	≥10 CESD No severe MDD (<7 MDD sx) on MINI	Life review combined with narrative therapy TAU	100 102	Group	CESD	Bsl Post tx 3 mo 9 mo (for LRT + NT only)	LRT sig better than TAU at post-tx and 3 mo Results maintained at 9 mo

Abbreviations: dx, diagnosis; MINI, The MINI Neuropsychiatric Interview; PRIME-MD, Primary Care Evaluation of Mental Disorders; sx, symptom.

symptoms were reported when comparing different types of CBT (ie, behavior therapy vs cognitive therapy, CBT group vs CBT Internet).

A total of 6 of the 8 CBT studies required a diagnosis of major depression, so it is difficult to determine if there were differences in efficacy depending on severity of depression. The 2 studies that included participants with subthreshold MDD used a more self-help approach (eg, bibliotherapy and Internet) to treatment. It would be interesting to know if self-help approaches would be as effective for participants with more severe depressive symptoms. In sum, CBT for late-life depression appears to be effective when compared with waitlist controls but is not superior to other forms of treatment.

Interpersonal Therapy

Interpersonal therapy (IPT) for depression was developed as a time-limited, structured treatment for depression and was based on the premise that depression onset and recurrence is related to an individual's interpersonal relationships at the time.[23,24] IPT focuses on current relationships in one (or more) of the following problem areas in the patient's life: grief, interpersonal conflict, role transitions, or interpersonal deficits. Techniques may include exploration, clarification, encouragement to express feelings, and behavior change techniques.[25] IPT has demonstrated efficacy for depression in general adult populations[26,27] and in combination with pharmacotherapy for late-life depression.[28,29] Less is known about IPT as a stand-alone treatment.

A total of 2 studies examining IPT met inclusion criteria for this review. van Schaik and colleagues[30] recruited patients from general medicine clinics with a diagnosis of MDD. Mossey and colleagues[31] used a modified version of IPT, called interpersonal counseling (IPC), to treat medically hospitalized patients with minor depression shortly after their discharge. In both studies, IPT and TAU were equally effective on measures of depression severity posttreatment. However, at 6-month follow-up, both studies reported significantly more improvement in the IPT/IPC groups compared with TAU. Thus, although IPT has strong support in the general adult depression literature, its effectiveness as a stand-alone treatment for late-life depression needs further research.

Problem-Solving Therapy

Problem-solving therapy (PST) is a form of CBT that focuses on teaching problem solving to prevent and reduce psychological distress.[32] Treatment involves teaching the patient to identify problems, brainstorm solutions, decide on a solution, implement the solution, and then evaluate whether it was effective. These skills can be taught in group or individual formats. PST has demonstrated efficacy across a wide range of populations, including adolescents and adults with diverse behavioral and physical disorders. A large meta-analysis examining PST for a range of physical and mental health problems indicated that PST was significantly more effective than no treatment, attention control, and TAU, and was as effective as other psychological treatments.[33] In two meta-analyses looking only at depression outcomes, similar results were reported in adolescents and adults.[34,35]

A total of 5 studies examining PST in late-life depression met criteria for this review and included individuals with MDD, MDD and executive dysfunction, minor depression, or dysthymia who were treated in a variety of settings including community and primary care clinics, and home health care. In all studies, participants were excluded if they were taking antidepressants. Among 7 comparison groups, PST demonstrated significant reductions in late-life depressive symptoms compared with waitlist control,[36] TAU,[37] reminiscence therapy,[36] supportive therapy,[38] and community-based psychotherapy.[39] A brief version of PST, PST-PC, was not more efficacious than paroxetine or placebo in a large study conducted in the primary care setting.[40] The investigators noted that there was significant site variability related to therapist skill and experience, which may have led to the negative results. Additionally, this version of PST has been criticized for being too brief (4–6 sessions) and not properly adapted for older adults.[41] PST appears to be effective for late-life depression, including older adults with depression and executive dysfunction.[38]

Reminiscence and Life Review

Reminiscence and life review interventions are based on Erikson's[42] last stage of life span development entitled "reflection on life." It was developed specifically for older adults and was first introduced as a therapeutic intervention in the 1970s.[43] Reminiscence interventions include simple or unstructured reminiscence, structured reminiscence or life review, and life review therapy or reminiscence therapy. Simple or unstructured reminiscence is essentially storytelling of life events with the goal of focusing on positive past events and enhancing well-being. Structured life review or reminiscence typically covers the entire life span and is more than just describing past events. It focuses on evaluating positive and negative events with the goal of reframing and integrating these events. Life review therapy is used with individuals who have clinically significant mental health problems, with the goal of changing one's view of themselves and the events in their life.

Reminiscence interventions have focused on a broad range of outcomes, including cognitive functioning, life satisfaction, and depression. In general, reminiscence has a moderate impact on psychological well-being in the general adult population, regardless of the presence of depression.[44,45] With regard to late-life depression, moderate effect sizes have been reported in meta-analyses.[44,46] However, it is frequently noted that there is significant heterogeneity in how the intervention is applied and that many of the studies in this area are of poor quality,[46] which may be related to a lag in theory development.[47]

A total of 4 studies examining reminiscence and life review therapy met criteria for this review. The studies included individuals with moderate to severe depressive symptoms who were recruited from a social service program[48] or from the community.[36,49,50] Life review therapy and reminiscence therapy were effective depression interventions when compared with no-treatment/attention control,[36,50] and TAU.[48,49] Structured reminiscence therapy had significantly greater improvement than unstructured reminiscence therapy on the Beck Depression Inventory (BDI),[50] but when compared with problem-solving therapy, it was less effective on 2 of 3 depression measures and had significantly lower rates of remission from depression at posttreatment (89% vs 40%).[36] All 4 studies used very different methods of reminiscence, rendering comparison difficult. In sum, reminiscence and life review therapy appear to be effective for late-life depressive symptoms but further research is required to determine what type of reminiscence therapy is most effective with a particular emphasis on developing a more structured treatment methodology.

Brief Psychodynamic Therapy

In treatments for late-life depression, brief psychodynamic therapy (BPD) has been examined only as a comparison group for CBT.[20,21] As discussed in the CBT section, BPD was better than waitlist control at posttreatment and equally effective compared with CBT in older adults recruited from the community.[20] These results were also maintained at 2-year follow-up.[51] Following the results of these studies, the investigators became more interested in BPD since meta-analyses at the time had typically reported that this form of therapy is generally not as effective as other therapies. They then conducted another study examining BPD and again compared it with CBT, but in a depressed caregiver group.[21] This brief psychodynamic therapy focused on 1 of the 4 following themes: independence, activity, self-esteem, or grief, and was based on the theory that caregivers past conflicts with their elderly relative are reactivated in the caregiving situation and lead to difficulty with separating ones own emotions and needs from those of their relative. Results of this study indicated, again, that there were no differences between CBT and BPD in reducing depressive symptoms; however, there was an interaction effect in that those individuals who had been caregivers for fewer than 3.5 years had more improvement in depression with BPD, whereas those with longer periods of caregiving had more improvement with CBT. The investigators hypothesized that coping resources may be depleted in long-term caregivers and that CBT provides very structured skills that assist in managing the stressor compared with processing the loss that they may be experiencing. To our knowledge, no studies of BPD in late-life depression (that met our inclusion criteria) have been conducted since the studies reported here. Thus, whereas the data indicate that it may be an effective treatment, further research is required.

DISCUSSION

Consistent with prior reviews and meta-analyses, the results indicate that psychological interventions are effective for the treatment of late-life depression. A total of 17 randomized studies examining CBT, PST, IPT, reminiscence therapy (RT), and BPD were evaluated and all therapies resulted in reduction of depressive symptoms. Given that older adults are generally accepting of psychological treatments,[7,8] it is promising that there are a variety of interventions to choose from. Not only was there a range of theoretical orientations, but the interventions spanned group, self-help, and individual treatments, which is consistent with the general adult population. From a clinical standpoint, this heterogeneity is positive, as it suggests there is flexibility in how to approach depression treatment for older adults. However, further research is needed to understand which of these treatments will work best for whom, particularly with regard to moderators such as age, depression severity, medical illness, or cognitive impairment.

The US population of individuals older than 65 is growing and it is estimated that 10% of this group will be age 90 and older by 2050, which is up from 4.7% in 2010. There are limited data on how to treat depression in the oldest old (age 85 and older) age group and they are the most likely to have chronic health conditions, cognitive impairment, and disability. A total of 20% to 30% of those who are age 90 or older live in nursing homes.[52] No studies in this review examined age as a moderator of treatment (see Ref[38] for exception) and we know very little about late-life depression in this oldest old group of adults. Two studies in this review conducted home-based treatments for those with medical disability but none examined interventions in residential facilities. Previous research not included in this review (due to sample size)[53,54] reported positive results for behavioral treatment targeting depression in nursing home residents. With regard to cognitive impairment, one study in this review specifically examined depression and cognitive dysfunction and it was concluded that modified PST was effective for this population.[38] These results are promising, but improved understanding of how to deliver psychological interventions outside of the traditional mental health setting and for those with comorbid medical illness and cognitive impairment is imperative.

Another important area of study is understanding how late-life depression severity moderates treatment outcome with specific attention as to how psychological treatments compare with or enhance pharmacologic treatment. Evidence-based guidelines recommend antidepressants and psychotherapy as the first-line treatment,[5] yet few studies outside of the IPT literature[29,55] have examined these in combination. In our review, 2 studies directly compared psychological interventions to medication with mixed results.[22,40]

Finally, although it is helpful to know that there are a variety of treatments that are effective for older adults, very little is known about how or why they work. In fact, the psychotherapy literature as a whole is lacking in understanding underlying mechanisms of change.[56] One approach, although controversial,[57] to explaining the lack of difference across multiple treatments that presumably differ in theory and technique is to consider the role of common factors, such as treatment alliance, expectations, education, and supportive environment. To our knowledge, there is no research on these factors in older adults, which is not surprising given the early stages of the research in this area.

Continued work in the area of psychological interventions for late-life depression is going to be dependent on having geriatric mental health specialists. There are concerns about whether the mental health care workforce is going to be prepared to work with older adults, and psychology in particular has not been as involved in geriatric policy, research, and clinical care.[58] A recent work group was convened to develop programs to recruit and retain geriatric mental health researchers.[59] Thus, there are movements at work to bridge the gap between a growing cohort of older adults and researchers specializing in late-life mental health.

CLINICAL VIGNETTE DEMONSTRATING USE OF CBT

SD is a 65-year-old, married White male self-referred for depression secondary to unemployment. He reported a long-standing history of dysthymia that was exacerbated over the past 2 years by his current unemployment status. He had received supportive treatment for nearly 10 years before presenting to our clinic and was unfamiliar with CBT. At the time of evaluation, his BDI score was 25 and he met criteria for MDD. He endorsed the following symptoms: depressed mood, anhedonia, fatigue, reduced appetite, sleep disturbance, impaired attention and concentration, and feelings of worthlessness and guilt. He denied current or past suicidal ideation. He engaged in significant rumination about his inability to obtain employment and fears that he and his wife were going to be poor and unable to enjoy retirement. Although his wife was supportive of the fact that he was unemployed, she was frustrated with his lack of engagement in the relationship and avoidance of responsibilities in the home.

Following the first session, SD was asked to monitor his activity level and it quickly became apparent that he was engaging in little activity other than watching TV, looking for jobs on the Internet, and reading news stories about the economy. He had previously enjoyed reading, socializing, cooking, travel, and participating in community activities with his wife. He cited finances as a reason for not doing these things and stated that he felt guilty spending money even though they had some income because his wife was still employed.

Psychoeducation was provided regarding the relationship between depressed mood and reduced activity. Treatment started with increasing his pleasurable activities and limiting his job search time each day to a specified time. SD's initial task was to cook a meal and was soon cooking several times a week. He stated that he felt a sense of satisfaction and being worthwhile and even began to enjoy seeking bargains and being creative to keep his expenses down. SD was also avoiding home maintenance and improvement tasks, such as cleaning and painting. These tasks were prioritized in session, broken down into smaller pieces and scheduled into his daily activities. Other behavioral techniques were used, including limiting computer time to specified hours and reducing daytime napping.

SD's endorsed beliefs, such as "I'm worthless without a job," "I feel guilty for enjoying myself when I should be working," and "I'm too old, no one will hire someone my age." Additionally, he would experience significant anxiety when getting a bill in the mail thinking "I can't afford this" and "I'm never going to enjoy retirement." Subsequent sessions were spent examining this belief and using cognitive therapy techniques, including thought records, identifying distortions, use of Socratic questions in session (eg, What would you think about a friend who didn't have a job), and use of cognitive restructuring. SD had more difficulty with the cognitive techniques and most of the treatment session focused on these beliefs.

After 20 sessions, SD still had not found a job but his BDI was reduced to a 4. He stated he was able to live his life in a manner that brought him pleasure without "beating up on himself" for being unemployed.

REFERENCES

1. Byers AL, Yaffe K, Covinsky KE, et al. High occurrence of mood and anxiety disorders among older adults: The National Comorbidity Survey Replication. Arch Gen Psychiatry 2010;67(5):489–96.
2. Blazer DG. Depression in late life: review and commentary. J Gerontol A Biol Sci Med Sci 2003;58(3):249–65.
3. Unutzer J, Katon W, Callahan CM, et al. Depression treatment in a sample of 1,801 depressed older adults in primary care. J Am Geriatr Soc 2003;51(4): 505–14.
4. Teresi J, Abrams R, Holmes D, et al. Prevalence of depression and depression recognition in nursing homes. Soc Psychiatry Psychiatr Epidemiol 2001;36(12): 613–20.
5. Shanmugham B, Karp J, Drayer R, et al. Evidence-based pharmacologic interventions for geriatric depression. Psychiatr Clin North Am 2005;28(4):821–35, viii.
6. Colenda CC, Wagenaar DB, Mickus M, et al. Comparing clinical practice with guideline recommendations for the treatment of depression in geriatric patients: findings from the APA practice research network. Am J Geriatr Psychiatry 2003; 11(4):448–57.
7. Landreville P, Landry J, Baillargeon L, et al. Older adults' acceptance of psychological and pharmacological treatments for depression. J Gerontol B Psychol Sci Soc Sci 2001;56(5):P285–91.
8. Gum AM, Arean PA, Hunkeler E, et al. Depression treatment preferences in older primary care patients. Gerontologist 2006;46(1):14–22.
9. Pinquart M, Duberstein PR, Lyness JM. Treatments for later-life depressive conditions: a meta-analytic comparison of pharmacotherapy and psychotherapy. Am J Psychiatry 2006;163(9):1493–501.
10. Butler AC, Chapman JE, Forman EM, et al. The empirical status of cognitive-behavioral therapy: a review of meta-analyses. Clin Psychol Rev 2006;26(1): 17–31.
11. Beck A. Cognitive therapy and the emotional disorders. Oxford (England): International Universities Press; 1976.
12. Lewinsohn P. A behavioral approach to depression. In: Friedman RJ, Katz MM, editors. The psychology of depression: contemporary theory and research. New York: Wiley; 1974. p. 157–85.
13. Pinquart M, Duberstein PR, Lyness JM. Effects of psychotherapy and other behavioral interventions on clinically depressed older adults: a meta-analysis. Aging Ment Health 2007;11(6):645–57.

14. Gould RL, Coulson MC, Howard RJ. Cognitive behavioral therapy for depression in older people: a meta-analysis and meta-regression of randomized controlled trials. J Am Geriatr Soc 2012;60(10):1817–30.
15. Wilson KC, Mottram PG, Vassilas CA. Psychotherapeutic treatments for older depressed people. Cochrane Database Syst Rev 2008;(1):CD004853.
16. Scogin F, Jamison C, Gochneaur K. Comparative efficacy of cognitive and behavioral bibliotherapy for mildly and moderately depressed older adults. J Consult Clin Psychol 1989;57(3):403–7.
17. Strachowski D, Khaylis A, Conrad A, et al. The effects of cognitive behavior therapy on depression in older patients with cardiovascular risk. Depress Anxiety 2008;25(8):E1–10.
18. Laidlaw K, Davidson K, Toner H, et al. A randomised controlled trial of cognitive behaviour therapy vs treatment as usual in the treatment of mild to moderate late life depression. Int J Geriatr Psychiatry 2008;23(8):843–50.
19. Serfaty MA, Haworth D, Blanchard M, et al. Clinical effectiveness of individual cognitive behavioral therapy for depressed older people in primary care: a randomized controlled trial. Arch Gen Psychiatry 2009;66(12):1332–40.
20. Thompson LW, Gallagher D, Breckenridge JS. Comparative effectiveness of psychotherapies for depressed elders. J Consult Clin Psychol 1987;55(3): 385–90.
21. Gallagher-Thompson D, Steffen AM. Comparative effects of cognitive-behavioral and brief psychodynamic psychotherapies for depressed family caregivers. J Consult Clin Psychol 1994;62(3):543–9.
22. Thompson LW, Coon DW, Gallagher-Thompson D, et al. Comparison of desipramine and cognitive/behavioral therapy in the treatment of elderly outpatients with mild-to-moderate depression. Am J Geriatr Psychiatry 2001;9(3):225–40.
23. Markowitz JC, Weissman MM. Interpersonal psychotherapy: past, present and future. Clin Psychol Psychother 2012;19(2):99–105.
24. Klerman G, Weissman M, Rounsaville B, et al. Interpersonal psychotherapy of depression. New York: Basic; 1984.
25. Hinrichsen G. Interpersonal psychotherapy as a treatment for late-life depression. In: Laidlaw K, Knight B, editors. Handbook of emotional disorders in later life. New York: Oxford University Press; 2008. p. 141–64.
26. de Mello MF, de Jesus Mari J, Bacaltchuk J, et al. A systematic review of research findings on the efficacy of interpersonal therapy for depressive disorders. Eur Arch Psychiatry Clin Neurosci 2005;255(2):75–82.
27. Cuijpers P, Geraedts AS, van Oppen P, et al. Interpersonal psychotherapy for depression: a meta-analysis. Am J Psychiatry 2011;168(6):581–92.
28. Reynolds CF 3rd, Dew MA, Pollock BG, et al. Maintenance treatment of major depression in old age. N Engl J Med 2006;354(11):1130–8.
29. Reynolds CF 3rd, Frank E, Perel JM, et al. Nortriptyline and interpersonal psychotherapy as maintenance therapies for recurrent major depression: a randomized controlled trial in patients older than 59 years. JAMA 1999;281(1): 39–45.
30. van Schaik A, van Marwijk H, Ader H, et al. Interpersonal psychotherapy for elderly patients in primary care. Am J Geriatr Psychiatry 2006;14(9):777–86.
31. Mossey JM, Knott KA, Higgins M, et al. Effectiveness of a psychosocial intervention, interpersonal counseling, for subdysthymic depression in medically ill elderly. J Gerontol A Biol Sci Med Sci 1996;51(4):M172–8.
32. D'Zurilla T, Nezu A. Problem-solving therapy: a social competence approach to clinical intervention. New York: Springer; 1999.

33. Malouff JM, Thorsteinsson EB, Schutte NS. The efficacy of problem solving therapy in reducing mental and physical health problems: a meta-analysis. Clin Psychol Rev 2007;27(1):46–57.

34. Bell AC, D'Zurilla TJ. Problem-solving therapy for depression: a meta-analysis. Clin Psychol Rev 2009;29(4):348–53.

35. Cuijpers P, Beekman A, Smit F, et al. Predicting the onset of major depressive disorder and dysthymia in older adults with subthreshold depression: a community based study. Int J Geriatr Psychiatry 2006;21(9):811–8.

36. Arean PA, Perri MG, Nezu AM, et al. Comparative effectiveness of social problem-solving therapy and reminiscence therapy as treatments for depression in older adults. J Consult Clin Psychol 1993;61(6):1003–10.

37. Gellis Z, McGinty J, Tierney L, et al. Randomized controlled trial of problem-solving therapy for minor depression in home care. Res Soc Work Pract 2008; 18:596–606.

38. Arean PA, Raue P, Mackin RS, et al. Problem-solving therapy and supportive therapy in older adults with major depression and executive dysfunction. Am J Psychiatry 2010;167(11):1391–8.

39. Arean P, Hegel M, Vannoy S, et al. Effectiveness of problem-solving therapy for older, primary care patients with depression: results from the IMPACT project. Gerontologist 2008;48(3):311–23.

40. Williams JW Jr, Barrett J, Oxman T, et al. Treatment of dysthymia and minor depression in primary care: a randomized controlled trial in older adults. JAMA 2000;284(12):1519–26.

41. Reynolds CF 3rd, Arean PA, Lynch TR, et al. Psychotherapy in old-age depression: progress and challenges. In: Roose S, Sackheim H, editors. Late-life depression. New York: Oxford University Press; 2004. p. 287–98.

42. Erikson E. Identity and the life cycle. New York: International University Press; 1959.

43. Butler R. The life-review: an interpretation of reminiscence in the aged. Psychiatry 1963;26:65–76.

44. Pinquart M, Forstmeier S. Effects of reminiscence interventions on psychosocial outcomes: a meta-analysis. Aging Ment Health 2012;16(5):541–58.

45. Bohlmeijer E, Roemer M, Cuijpers P, et al. The effects of reminiscence on psychological well-being in older adults: a meta-analysis. Aging Ment Health 2007; 11(3):291–300.

46. Bohlmeijer E, Smit F, Cuijpers P. Effects of reminiscence and life review on late-life depression: a meta-analysis. Int J Geriatr Psychiatry 2003;18(12):1088–94.

47. Westerhof G, Bohlmeijer E, Webster J. Reminiscence and mental health: a review of recent progress in theory, research and interventions. Ageing Soc 2010;30(4):697–721.

48. Serrano JP, Latorre JM, Gatz M, et al. Life review therapy using autobiographical retrieval practice for older adults with depressive symptomatology. Psychol Aging 2004;19(2):270–7.

49. Korte J, Bohlmeijer ET, Cappeliez P, et al. Life review therapy for older adults with moderate depressive symptomatology: a pragmatic randomized controlled trial. Psychol Med 2012;42(6):1163–73.

50. Fry P. Structured and unstructured reminiscence training and depression among the elderly. Clin Gerontologist 1983;1(3):15–37.

51. Gallagher-Thompson D, Hanley-Peterson P, Thompson LW. Maintenance of gains versus relapse following brief psychotherapy for depression. J Consult Clin Psychol 1990;58(3):371–4.

52. He W, Muenchrath M. 90+ in the United States: 2006–2008. Washington, DC: U.S. Government Printing Office; 2011.

53. Meeks S, Looney SW, Van Haitsma K, et al. BE-ACTIV: a staff-assisted behavioral intervention for depression in nursing homes. Gerontologist 2008;48(1): 105–14.

54. Teri L, Logsdon RG, Uomoto J, et al. Behavioral treatment of depression in dementia patients: a controlled clinical trial. J Gerontol B Psychol Sci Soc Sci 1997; 52(4):P159–66.

55. Reynolds CF 3rd, Dew MA, Martire LM, et al. Treating depression to remission in older adults: a controlled evaluation of combined escitalopram with interpersonal psychotherapy versus escitalopram with depression care management. Int J Geriatr Psychiatry 2010;25(11):1134–41.

56. Kazdin AE. Mediators and mechanisms of change in psychotherapy research. Annu Rev Clin Psychol 2007;3:1–27.

57. DeRubeis RJ, Brotman MA, Gibbons CJ. A conceptual and methodological analysis of the nonspecifics argument. Clin Psychol Sci Pract 2005;12(2): 174–83.

58. Karel MJ, Gatz M, Smyer MA. Aging and mental health in the decade ahead: what psychologists need to know. Am Psychol 2012;67(3):184–98.

59. Bartels SJ, Lebowitz BD, Reynolds CF 3rd, et al. Programs for developing the pipeline of early-career geriatric mental health researchers: outcomes and implications for other fields. Acad Med 2010;85(1):26–35.

What is the Role of Alternative Treatments in Late-life Depression?

Maren Nyer, PhD[a],*, James Doorley, BA[a], Kelley Durham, BA[a],
Albert S. Yeung, MD, ScD[a], Marlene P. Freeman, MD[b],
David Mischoulon, MD, PhD[a]

KEYWORDS

- Late-life depression • Natural remedies • Exercise • Yoga • Tai chi
- Massage therapy • Music therapy • Spirituality

KEY POINTS

- Many available CAM interventions show promise for elderly people with depression.
- Natural remedies have encouraging evidence of efficacy and safety and may be well suited to older people due to their more modest side-effect profiles than conventional medications have.
- Nonpharmacologic physical interventions, such as exercise, yoga, tai chi, and massage therapy, have demonstrated benefit in the elderly.
- Less physically oriented interventions, such as music therapy and spiritual-religious–based therapy, also have encouraging but preliminary evidence in their support.
- Research on CAM therapies in older populations is still limited, and more work is needed before clinicians know how best to recommend these interventions.

INTRODUCTION

Clinicians who treat elderly patients with depression need to be especially careful about several issues. First, older patients are particularly vulnerable to antidepressant side effects, such as gastrointestinal upset, sedation, and sexual dysfunction.[1] Second, older patients are often taking multiple prescription medications for medical conditions, increasing the risk of drug-drug interactions that may occur when psychotropic drugs are added to the pharmacologic mix. Third, many older patients may be resistant to taking antidepressants because of generational stigmas about mental

[a] Depression Clinical and Research Program, Department of Psychiatry, Massachusetts General Hospital, Harvard Medical School, 1 Bowdoin Square, 6th Floor, Boston, MA 02114, USA;
[b] Perinatal and Reproductive Psychiatry Program, Department of Psychiatry, Massachusetts General Hospital, Harvard Medical School, 185 Cambridge Street, 2nd Floor, Boston, MA 02114, USA
* Corresponding author.
E-mail address: mnyer@partners.org

Psychiatr Clin N Am 36 (2013) 577–596
http://dx.doi.org/10.1016/j.psc.2013.08.012
0193-953X/13/$ – see front matter © 2013 Elsevier Inc. All rights reserved.
psych.theclinics.com

Abbreviations: Alternative Treatments for Late-life Depression	
EPA	Eicosapentaenoic acid
DHA	Docosahexaenoic acid
CAM	Complementary and alternative medicine
SAMe	S-Adenosyl methionine
MDD	Major depressive disorder
TCA	Tricyclic antidepressant
SJW	St. John's Wort (Hypericum perforatum L.)
SSRI	Selective serotonin reuptake inhibitor
SNRI	Serotonin-norepinephrine reuptake inhibitor
5-MTHF	5-Methyltetrahydrofolate
HPA	Hypothalamic-pituitary-adrenal
RCT	Randomized clinical trial
CBT	Cognitive behavior therapy

illness and treatment.[2] The popularity of CAM has been growing over the past few decades, with increasing consumer use in the United States and worldwide,[3,4] among the general population as well as older adults.[5] CAM interventions, both pharmacologic and nonpharmacologic, may be desirable to older patients, in view of the decreased risk of side effects and drug-drug interactions.[6] This article reviews several popular CAM interventions that may be well suited to elderly patients.

NATURAL REMEDIES

Natural and nutritional supplements are among the most commonly used CAM therapies in the United States.[4] One major appeal of these natural products is their ease of access, because most can be obtained over the counter, without the need for prescription.[7] Research on these remedies has increased concurrently with their popularity. For a few CAM therapies, there is currently a reasonably large, although often ambiguous, body of data regarding their clinical efficacy, safety, and mechanisms of action. For others, however, data remain sparse.

Much of the research on CAM products has been conducted in general adult populations, typically consisting of men and women of ages 18 to 65. There are, unfortunately, fewer studies that have focused on the efficacy and safety of these therapies in older adults, and most of the existing studies have tended to focus on natural products that target dementia and insomnia, which are especially common problems in the elderly. Less investigation exists on mood-enhancing products in this demographic. This article focuses on some of the more widely used natural antidepressants and reviews evidence and implications for their use in the elderly.

St. John's Wort (Hypericum perforatum L.)

There are approximately 40 published clinical trials of SJW monotherapy for depression, with generally positive evidence, although recent meta-analyses have emphasized their overall mixed findings, particularly when considering newer studies that compare SJW against SSRIs.[8]

There is at least 1 published study of SJW focusing specifically on samples older than age 65. Harrer and colleagues[9] carried out a 6-week, randomized double-blind comparison of SJW (800 mg/d) against fluoxetine (20 mg/d) in 149 elderly patients with International Statistical Classification of Diseases, Tenth Revision mild or moderate depressive episodes. Both medications were well tolerated and similarly effective based on decrease in Hamilton Depression Rating Scale scores. A more recent study that included adults from ages 18 up to 70 with atypical depression also suggested medications benefit for SJW (600 mg/d) over placebo.[10]

Hyperforin, one of SJW's active ingredients, has been shown in animal models to decrease amyloid deposits, suggesting a potential antidementia effect.[11] This, and the generally good tolerability of SJW, suggests that it could be a good option for elderly people who may suffer from cognitive deficits and who may be especially prone to side effects from standard antidepressants. This would be an important focus of future research.

Of great clinical importance, SJW has been shown to have several interactions with other drugs via induction of the cytochrome P450 enzymes, CYP3A4 and CYP2C9,[6] and this is a significant concern when dealing with elderly patients who may already be taking many medications for various medical conditions. In particular, the combination of SJW with SSRIs has resulted in serotonin syndrome, a potentially fatal reaction.[6] For this reason, no patient should combine SJW with SSRIs. SJW can induce the metabolism of warfarin, some antiretrovirals, immunosuppresants, β-blockers, calcium channel blockers, atiarrhythmics (such as digoxin), and statins, among other medications.[6] SJW can also induce the metabolism of estrogens,[6] which may be clinically important in women on estrogen hormone therapy.

Recommended doses of SJW range from 900 mg/d to 1800 mg/d in adults, although the strength of different preparations may vary due to standardization based on the active ingredients. The best recommendation for the elderly is to use SJW only under physician supervision, begin at low doses, and be extremely mindful of potential interactions with other drugs.

Fish Oil

The omega-3 fatty acids, derived from fish oil, have also been extensively studied in mood disorders, with more than 30 published clinical trials, usually of combinations of EPA and DHA.[12–14] Studies seem to support antidepressant efficacy, both as monotherapy and as augmentation of standard antidepressants. A recent meta-analysis[13] found that preparations comprising EPA:DHA ratios of 3:2 or greater produced the most robust antidepressant effects. Recommended doses for depression based on these studies are approximately 1000 mg/d. There is at least 1 published clinical trial examining the omega-3 fatty acids in elderly depressed populations. Rondanelli and colleagues[15] carried out an 8-week, randomized, double-blind, placebo-controlled trial of an omega-3 preparation (2.5 g/d) against placebo in 46 depressed female nursing home residents, ages 66 to 95. The investigators found a significant improvement in depressive symptoms as well as in quality-of-life symptoms in the omega-3 group compared with the placebo group.

The recent Bloch and Hannestad[14] meta-analysis suggested minimal antidepressant benefit of omega-3 fatty acids in general adult samples and stated that much of its observed efficacy was likely attributable to publication bias. There was, however, some debate regarding the methods of this analysis.[16–18] The antidepressant efficacy of omega-3 fatty acids thus requires further clarification.

There is some promising evidence from 11 observational studies and 4 clinical trials that consumption of fish or omega-3 supplements may prevent or slow cognitive decline in the elderly but not prevent or treat dementia per se.[19] Omega-3s also have well documented benefits in cardiovascular and joint health,[12,20] two other potentially important indications for the elderly population. Finally, omega-3s seem to have limited interactions with other drugs, which makes them especially appealing for use with the elderly. There is a risk, however, of bleeding with higher doses and/or in combination with anticoagulants.[12] For this reason, the elderly should use omega-3s at doses of less than 3 g/d and never in combination with major anticoagulants, such as warfarin or heparin, without a physician's supervision.

S-Adenosyl Methionine

SAMe has approximately 45 clinical trials supporting efficacy, primarily for monotherapy of MDD.[21,22] Evidence for combination of SAMe with other agents is also encouraging, although limited. Two studies showed efficacy of the combination of SAMe plus a TCA,[23,24] and 2 studies, 1 open[25] and 2 placebo-controlled,[26] have shown benefit of SAMe augmentation for partial responders to SSRIs and SNRIs.

Doses of SAMe reported in the literature for treating depression are usually between 800 mg/d and 1600 mg/d, although higher doses are sometimes needed. Mild gastrointestinal upset is the most commonly reported side effect.[27] Care with dosing should be taken in elderly patients, and it is advisable to begin with low doses and increase gradually as tolerated. SAMe also seems to have beneficial effects on joint health,[27] another potential benefit for the elderly. There is also some limited evidence for SAMe having a positive impact on cognition in older adults.[28] Studies examining SAMe specifically in elderly populations are sorely lacking, although there is 1 open study suggesting antidepressant benefits in patients with Parkinson disease.[29] Overall, the apparent safety, tolerability, and lack of interactions suggest that SAMe may have a niche in the treatment of late-life depression and deserves further study.

Folic Acid

There has been a longstanding association between low folate and depression.[30] A few studies have examined several different folic acid forms as antidepressants, particularly in combination with standard agents, with encouraging results.[30,31] A recent study on 5-MTHF (Deplin) supports efficacy as an antidepressant adjunct at doses of 15 mg/d.[32] This form may be particularly effective because it crosses the blood-brain barrier directly and can in theory deliver more active product to where it is most needed.

Another potential role for folate supplementation is in prevention of dementia. A few studies suggest beneficial effects of folate supplementation for elderly patients with dementia or other memory deficits.[30] Homocysteine, a 1-carbon cycle metabolite, may be a contributor to dementia when present in excess. Because folate supplementation can reduce homocysteine, this too presents an argument for folate supplementation in the elderly.[30]

Because the elderly are often at risk of poor nutrition, supplementation with folate is generally a good idea in this demographic. Given the excellent tolerability of the various folate forms, regular use of folate in the elderly with or without depression seems called for. Folate seems to have no adverse interactions with other agents, which again makes it especially appealing in the elderly. Doses may vary depending on the specific folate form used.

Summary: Natural Supplements

The good tolerability of the reviewed natural products along with their encouraging evidence of efficacy suggests that there may be a place for them in the management of late-life depression. Care needs to be taken when combining SJW with standard medications, and in general, the conventional wisdom to start low and go slow applies. Likewise, patients with significant medical comorbidity need to be especially careful. Further research in older depressed populations is needed in order to better understand the potential benefits and liabilities of these products in this demographic. Finally, older adults as well as those of any age should be asked routinely about use of supplements and educated that "natural" does not always mean safe. Many commonly used CAM treatments remain largely unstudied and further research is encouraged.

EXERCISE

The overall health benefits of physical exercise have long been recognized and scientifically supported for a variety of populations.[33–35] Higher physical activity levels among older adults in particular may have a preventive effect on the development of depression.[36] Recent findings point to the potential efficacy of exercise as a treatment of depression in older adults, in some cases with similar efficacy to antidepressants.[37–39]

Although many previous studies have focused on younger adults, several studies have examined older adult samples. Some results suggest that exercise may be more useful in treating depressive symptoms among older adults than younger adults.[40] For example, Fukukawa and colleagues[41] assessed a community sample of Japanese men and women between 40 and 70 years of age. At 2-year follow-up, participation in exercise was predictive of a reduction in depressive symptoms for participants 65 years and older, and no significant association was found for middle-aged participants (ages 40–64). Results are not conclusive, however, regarding the long-term effects of exercise for depression, with some studies yielding nonsignificant differences between groups after 3-month to 6-month follow-up periods.[42–44]

Studies have individually examined both anaerobic and aerobic exercise for depressed older adults, with promising evidence for both.[45] A study by Singh and colleagues[46] yielded a 59% response rate (defined by a 50% reduction in the sum score of the Hamilton Depression Rating Scale) for older adults assigned to an anaerobic exercise condition compared with a 26% response rate for controls ($P = .067$). Aerobic exercise may be particularly useful in treating somatic symptoms of depression[47] and was found comparable with medications in reducing depressive symptoms in older adults with MDD.

The format of exercise (ie, supervised or unsupervised) may be an important variable to consider.[48,49] Timonen and colleagues[43] compared supervised anaerobic exercise (ie, strength training) twice a week with unsupervised home-based exercise 2 to 3 times per week. Depressive symptoms were significantly reduced ($P = .048$) for participants in the supervised exercise group compared with those in the unsupervised group, suggesting that either adherence to exercise regime, social support, or both may mediate the effects of exercise on depressive symptoms. Although this study used a walking intervention, Dunn and colleagues[50] reported that greater energy expenditure is associated with a greater decrease in depressive symptoms. Impact based on frequency and/or intensity of exercise should also be investigated, because exercise seems to have a dose-response effect.[39]

Several psychological and physiologic mechanisms have been proposed to explain the effects of exercise on late-life depression. Possible psychological factors include increased self-efficacy, distraction, an increased sense of mastery, and changes in self-concept.[51] Potential physiologic factors include increased levels of circulating β-endorphins and monoamines,[52,53] increased central norepinephrine neurotransmission along with serotonin synthesis and metabolism,[54–56] and improved quality of sleep, which is often disturbed in depression.[57]

Physical exercise may be effective in relieving symptoms of mild to moderate depression in older adults.[45,47,50] Despite the promising results of previous studies, methodological problems, such as small sample size, varying definitions of depression, and insufficient follow-up data, limit existing findings.[40] Further well-controlled studies are required comparing the effects of different forms of exercise on late-life depression.

YOGA

Yoga is an ancient mind-body practice originating from India that promotes certain philosophic life values and spiritual, physical, and emotional health. Yoga practices typically focus on physical postures, breathing, meditation, and spiritual philosophy. There are many styles of yoga practiced in the United States, ranging from more gentle to vigorous and also varying in degree of spiritual focus.[58] For the elderly or those who have physical limitations, yoga-based intervention may need to be gentler. Spiritual interventions show promise in this population (discussed later), so this aspect may appeal to this cohort. Alternatively, Eastern philosophic ideas may not be as well received due to generational issues.

The popularity of yoga in the Untied States has increased in recent years. Yoga is broadly practiced in the United States: 10.4 million individuals in the United States practiced yoga in the past 12 months in 2002. Of those, 20% used yoga for mental health purposes and 75% found it helpful.[59] Following the public interest, the scientific literature base of yoga has substantially increased in recent years. Further scientific understanding of the benefits of yoga may encourage integration of yoga as a medical intervention into Western medicine for the elderly. For example, physician recommendation, public health programming, and insurance reimbursement may follow empiric validation, allowing marginalized populations access to the modality, such as those who are late in life.

Yoga and Health

Research demonstrating yoga's broad-reaching implications for promoting wellness and managing and treating chronic conditions is growing. In a recent literature review of normal aged adults, yoga resulted in improvement of multiple markers of physical health.[60] Yoga has demonstrated improvements in quality of life in people with various conditions (ie, rheumatoid arthritis,[61] atrial fibrillation,[62] chronic neck pain,[63] asthma in women,[64] cancer survivors hip,[65] pain,[66] and distress in women).[67] Because these conditions are more common in later life, yoga may be a particularly viable mind-body intervention for these individuals.

Yoga has demonstrated benefits to health in those in late life. In a meta-analysis of older adults, yoga may hold greater benefits than conventional exercise for health status, aerobic fitness, and strength.[68] Yoga has also shown benefit in older adults with obesity and type 2 diabetes mellitus with regard to improvement in overall physical function and capacity, reduced stress and anxiety, enhanced calmness, and improved sleep quality and efforts toward dietary improvements.[69] These data suggest that yoga may be useful not only for managing chronic illness in older adults but also for simultaneously improving mood and sleep—both important in the treatment of depression. Yoga demonstrates great promise as an intervention for both illness, common in the elderly, and mood/depression.

Yoga and Depression

There is mounting evidence that different forms of yoga work to treat symptoms of depression, although the majority of studies suffer from methodological limitations.[70,71] There is limited evidence to suggest that yoga is effective in late-life depression. In a 3-armed study, 69 older adults (aged 60+), living in a residential care facility in India, were randomized to a 24-week yoga (ie, postures, relaxation, and spiritual aspects), ayurveda (ie, herbal preparation), or a wait-list condition. Participants were not selected for depression, although geriatric depression was the primary outcome measure. The yoga group was the only group to show substantial decreases in geriatric depression scores at 3 months and 6 months; however, the design did not adequately control for the time spent with the yoga group (7.5 hours per week).[72]

Depression is frequently associated with cognitive impairments, which may be associated with other sources of functional impairment.[73] Yoga has shown the ability to improve concentration and cognitive functioning in healthy adults.[74] This effect may occur through deep focus on breathing and muscle movement.[75] The reduction of stress, anxiety, and depression, in addition to physiologic regulation of the stress response system, may also improve cognitive function, an area of particular importance to the elderly.

Yoga may improve depression in the elderly through various methods, including mindfulness and exercise (discussed in sections on Exercise and Tai Chi). Yoga may also help alleviate symptoms of medical conditions that are often comorbid with depression, especially in the elderly (eg, pain, hypertension, and musculoskeletal symptoms). Depression is closely linked to the body's physiologic reaction to stress.[76] Yoga has consistently demonstrated the ability to decrease perceived levels of stress[77] and physiologic markers of the stress response system in many different populations.[77–84] Many chronic diseases are related to the stress response system, which again suggests that yoga is well suited to simultaneously treat medical and psychiatric comorbidities. Finally, benefits on sleep may also have a positive impact on mood. The vicious cycle of sleep disturbance increasing depressive symptoms and depressive symptoms worsening sleep creates a self-reinforcing pattern. Yoga may act synergistically to improve mood directly and indirectly by simultaneously improving sleep. Improved sleep regulation may be a mechanism of action for yoga's antidepressant effects, perhaps via improved sleep efficiency and quality.[70] Yoga has demonstrated benefits for sleep disturbance in older adults in a few preliminary trials.[85]

Summary: Yoga

Yoga has demonstrated preliminary evidence for the treatment of depression in general adult and older populations. The research base, however, is still in its infancy. Evidence is mounting for yoga's ability to treat medical comorbidities frequently seen in the elderly, in addition to improving physical functioning. Because of the synergy of exercise, physiologic benefits, and mindfulness, in addition to ease of implementation of yoga-based interventions, yoga is a promising area of treatment of elderly depression, and an important area for future research.

TAI CHI

Tai chi (or t'ai chi ch'uan) is originally a form of martial art developed in ancient China. It is now mostly practiced as a graceful form of mind-body exercise and is growing in popularity in the West. Recent data from the National Health Interview Survey suggest that approximately 5 million Americans have practiced tai chi and that this number is increasing.[86,87] Tai chi involves a series of gentle movements, often coordinated with breathing and imagery, that aim to strengthen and relax the physical body and mind, enhance the natural flow of *qi* (life energy), and improve health and personal development.[88]

In tai chi, each posture flows into the next without pause, ensuring that the body is in constant motion, which promotes a sense of serenity. Through a self-paced system of gentle physical exercise and stretching, body awareness, and breath regulation, tai chi is considered meditation in motion. There are many different tai chi styles. Each style may have its own subtle emphasis on various tai chi principles and methods. The advantage of tai chi is that it is low impact and puts minimal stress on muscles and joints, making it generally safe for people of all ages and fitness levels. It is particularly beneficial for older adults who otherwise may not exercise. In addition, it is inexpensive, requires no special equipment, and can be done in or outdoors, either alone or in a group.

Tai Chi and Health

Tai chi shows great potential for becoming widely integrated into initiatives related to the prevention and rehabilitation of several medical conditions, including mental health. A growing body of clinical research has begun to evaluate the efficacy of tai chi as a therapy for a variety of health issues, including coronary artery disease,[89] heart failure,[90] hypertension[91] and general cardiorespiratory fitness,[92] balance and postural stability,[93] musculoskeletal strength and flexibility,[94] multiple sclerosis,[95] rheumatoid arthritis,[96] osteoarthritis,[97] microcirculation and endothelial function,[98] and immune function.[99] Several tai chi review articles have been published suggesting varied health benefits in various areas.[100–102] Preliminary research has shown tai chi's beneficial effects on a range of psychological well-being measures, including mood, anxiety, general stress management, self-esteem, and quality of life in varied populations.[103]

Tai Chi and Depression

In a systematic review, Wang and colleagues[104] reviewed studies published in either Chinese or English and concluded that tai chi exercises seem to be associated with improvements in psychological well-being, including reduced stress, anxiety, and depression. Subjects in most of the studies cited in this review, however, were recruited for tai chi intervention based on their medical conditions, including osteoarthritis and obesity, and improvements in depression were secondary outcomes.

Only a few studies have evaluated tai chi specifically for patients with depression or clearly defined MDD. Thirty-nine Chinese Americans with moderate to moderately severe MDD were randomized into a 12-week tai chi intervention or a wait-listed control group in a 2:1 ratio. The tai chi intervention group, compared with the control group, had improved response rate (21% vs 0%) and remission rate (19% vs 0%), although the difference did not reach statistical significance. No adverse events were reported.[105]

There are 2 published studies of tai chi offered to elderly patients with depression. Chou and colleagues[106] reported a small randomized controlled trial of 14 older Chinese patients with depression, suggesting beneficial impact of tai chi on 5 measures of depressive symptoms (ie, the Center For Epidemiologic Studies Depression Scale total score and 4 subscale scores—somatic symptoms, negative affects, interpersonal relations, and well-being). Lavretsky and colleagues[107] studied older adults with MDD who were partial responders to antidepressants. The results showed that participants who received tai chi had greater reductions in depressive symptoms, greater improvement in physical functioning, and decreased inflammatory markers compared with the health education control group. They concluded that tai chi might provide additional improvements of clinical outcomes in the pharmacologic treatment of geriatric depression.

The practice of tai chi is an excellent way to train body relaxation and mindfulness, which could reduce depression through several possible mechanisms. In a series of studies, Benson and colleagues[108] demonstrated that the "relaxation response," a form of meditation that uses a set of simple instructions, results in measurable, predictable, and reproducible physiologic changes that include reductions in oxygen consumption, carbon dioxide production, respiratory rate, blood pressure, and arterial blood lactate.[109]

The ability to relax the body through tai chi training could attenuate the stress response from the HPA axis, which has been hypothesized to be involved in the neurobiology of clinical depression, panic symptoms, and posttraumatic stress disorder.[110-112] From a psychological perspective, tai chi and other meditation practices could have a variety of potential therapeutic effects, including exposure, desensitization, deautomatization, catharsis, and counterconditioning.[113] Other investigators have mentioned gain of insight, self-monitoring, self-control, and self-understanding as outcomes.[114]

Two psychological mechanisms that may be especially important in understanding how meditation may be helpful for depression are enhanced regulation of attention and disidentification with negative thoughts.[115] Tai chi, like other forms of meditation, has the goal of helping practitioners better regulate their attention and reduce ruminative preoccupation. People who meditate suspend their habits of judging and interpreting by not focusing their attention on the outside world and by attending to the present moment without allowing themselves to be distracted by anxieties, fantasies, and memories.[116] In this regard, tai chi can be viewed as a systematic way of regulating attention.

The second process is disidentification with negative thoughts, the method whereby the mind only observes and ceases to identify with mental content, such as thoughts, feelings, and images.[115] The heightened awareness brought about by tai chi and other forms of meditation allows practitioners to recognize and disidentify thoughts and emotions and to observe all experiences with calmness and equanimity. Practitioners can do this because they have developed a tranquil state of mind, which has variously been described as "transcendental consciousness," "Zen," and "divine apathy," among other terms.[116]

Summary: Tai Chi

There are few studies on the use of tai chi for treatment of depression among older adults, and many of the studies recruited patients with medical conditions, not MDD. The existing evidence suggests possible benefits from the use of tai chi for treatment of older adults with depression. Future studies are needed to target older adults with MDD and explore therapeutic elements of tai chi in treating depression in older adults.

MASSAGE THERAPY

Massage therapy is a popular intervention for many physical and psychological concerns. It involves direct manipulation of the muscles, including rubbing, kneading, brushing, and tapping in selected bodily locations.[8] The main purpose of massage is to induce release of physical and emotional tension. Although some clinical trials have examined massage in general adult populations with anxious, depressive, and stress-related symptoms,[8] there are few published studies on massage therapy in older adults.

Hirakawa and colleagues[117] carried out a study of home massage rehabilitation therapy in bed-ridden elderly patients in which no mental or physical positive effects were found. Sharpe and associates,[118] however, reported positive results in a study in which patients were assigned to massage versus guided relaxation. Subjects who received massage experienced significant improvement in anxiety, depression, vitality, general health, and positive well-being compared with patients in the guided relaxation group.

Regarding tolerability, in a prospective study of side effects in 100 adult massage participants, 10% of subjects reported minor post-treatment discomforts, usually beginning within 12 hours of the massage session and persisting for less than 36 hours. Alternatively, 23% of participants reported nonmusculoskeletal positive effects, usually starting right after the massage session and persisting for more than 48 hours.[119] It remains unclear whether tolerability would be comparable among older populations.

Although massage therapy is appealing in view of its benign and nonpharmacologic nature, research is limited, and more studies are needed before clinicians can know how best to recommend this intervention to elderly patients with depression. Because massage therapy is a highly unregulated industry,[8] with varying certification standards from state to state, individuals who are interested in this modality need to be careful to ensure that their therapist has the proper qualifications.

MUSIC THERAPY

A few studies have been published measuring the efficacy of music therapy for late-life depression. The interventions used in these studies can be broadly classified either as active, in which a patient recreates, improvises, or composes music, or as receptive, in which a patient listens to music.[120] Music therapy was first reported as an effective treatment of depressive symptoms by Hadsell[121] and Benenzon[122] and may be particularly effective in helping depressed older adults express their emotions.[123]

Subsequent RCTs have suggested potential benefits for late-life depression. One study compared therapist-delivered music therapy to independent, home-based music therapy exercises in a sample of depressed older adults. Results showed that independent, home-based exercises were more effective in reducing depressive symptoms.[124] Alternatively, Zerhusen and colleagues[125] found group music therapy to be less effective than group CBT for depressed older adults. The configuration of the 2 groups differed in both length of session and number of participants, raising questions regarding the structural integrity and, subsequently, the utility of the music therapy intervention used.[126]

Music therapy may also be effective for older depressed adults taking antidepressant medications. Chen[127] found that the combination of antidepressants with active music therapy was more effective than antidepressants alone. Subjects in the augmentation group showed improvement within the first week on average, whereas those taking antidepressants alone did not show improvement until the 3rd or 4th week. Also, dropout rates in these studies were low, with 1 study reporting no dropouts.[127] This study suggests a potential advantage of adjunctive music therapy for treating late-life depression.

Of the existing RCTs, several point to potential benefits of music therapy for late-life depression. Possible mechanisms of action may include the creation of new aesthetic, physical, and relational experiences through active music making in a supportive collaboration between patient and therapist.[128] Music may also provide depressed older adults with a more comfortable alternative for expressing emotion, which may be particularly challenging for this population.[126] Still, many studies have suffered from small sample sizes, heterogeneous participant groups, and overall low methodological quality.[126] Further research is needed to differentiate the effects of different forms of music therapy on late-life depression.

RELIGION AND SPIRITUALITY

Religion and spirituality–based interventions may be viable treatments for depression in older adults. Many older adults value religion and spirituality, and religious beliefs are particularly notable in older adults as well as in individuals with chronic illnesses.[129] According to a survey, 77% to 83% of older adult participants prefer to include spirituality in their treatment, although the sample of this study was primarily Christian.[129]

A recent review reported that no spiritual or religious treatment had been established for older adults.[130] The development of such treatments is important, considering not only older adults' preferences for incorporating these beliefs but also their overall preference for behavioral over psychopharmacologic treatments and the high occurrence of depressive symptoms in this population.[131]

Although few studies have specifically evaluated religious and spiritual interventions in older adults, there is evidence to support further research. Religion and spirituality can be protective factors against mental illness[132] as well as helpful coping mechanisms.[133] Several studies have also shown that incorporation of religion and spirituality into already established treatments can be beneficial.[134] Religious and spiritual practices have goals similar to those of psychotherapy. For example, both emphasize the search for identity and meaning as well as themes such as optimism and coping. Both attempt to create a framework with which to understand human experiences. As a result, religion and spirituality can effectively work in conjunction with psychotherapy.

In a review of religious and spiritual therapies, several studies evaluated Christian accommodative cognitive therapy.[135] These interventions provided cognitive therapy in a religious or spiritual context by using the Bible and religious imagery. All these studies showed that the religious intervention was more effective than various control interventions, such as supportive therapies and secular therapies, and at least as effective as pharmacologic therapies, such as antidepressants and anxiolytics. A few studies examined Muslim psychotherapy for depression when used in conjunction with standard psychotherapy and medication. It is difficult to determine if the positive results of these studies are due to the effectiveness of the established secular treatment or if the religious elements are enhancing the treatment. It seems that with regard to these therapies, appropriate matching of patients to therapy is of prime importance.

One study from the aforementioned review[136] is still frequently cited as an example of incorporation of religion and spirituality into CBT. Religious participants were assigned to 3 different groups: religious CBT (including religious content as part of the therapy), nonreligious CBT, and pastoral care therapy. Every participant completed 18 50-minute sessions and both CBT groups participated in cognitive restructuring and homework assignments. Individuals who received the religious CBT experienced a greater decrease in depressive symptoms than those in the nonreligious CBT.

There are fewer studies that examined interventions specifically developed to address religion and spirituality. Moritz and colleagues[132] tested the effectiveness of an 8-week home study–based religion and spirituality education program for mood disturbance (based on score of >40 on the Profile of Mood States). Participants in the religion and spirituality program were compared with participants in a mindfulness-based stress reduction class and a to wait-list control group. Those in the religion and spirituality education class received audiotapes with the week's lesson and a visualization exercise for daily use. The education program was as effective as other interventions and specifically effective for depressive symptoms. Participants in the religious and spiritual education program showed greater improvement in mood and higher compliance than those in the mindfulness-based stress reduction group.

Another study examined the treatment of minor depression and subsyndromal anxiety in older adults,[131] using an intervention involving a prayer wheel created by Rossiter-Thornton.[137] The prayer wheel, which is nondenominational and standardized, consists of 8 5-minute exercises. Rajagopal and associates[131] compared participants using the prayer wheel individually with participants using the prayer wheel as a group. The group experienced a trend in decreased depressive symptoms. Although no change was seen in those participants using the wheel individually, participants who continued to use the wheel after the study were significantly less depressed at follow-up compared with those who did not. Therefore, the intervention may be more effective after a longer period of implementation.

When using any of the aforementioned religious and spiritual treatments for older adults, there are several factors to consider.[133] First, a person's motivation for religious and spiritual beliefs or practices is important. If a person is intrinsically motivated, religious practices can contribute to positive health outcomes. If a person is externally motivated by rewards, however, such as social status, religious practices can contribute to negative health outcomes. Furthermore, people who use religion to rationalize stressful life events in a positive way and believe they can become stronger from such experiences often have more positive health outcomes, whereas those who view stressful life events as punishment or a result of personal shortcomings often have negative health outcomes. Finally, it is important to determine if a person perceives treatment to be in conflict with religious or spiritual beliefs. For example, a person may believe that seeking treatment is wrong or interferes with God's plan. All these factors should be considered to assess whether including religious or spiritual components helps or hinders treatment.

Research on religious and spiritual interventions for depression is limited, especially within the older adult population. Further research should be conducted on incorporating religious and spiritual elements into established treatments as well as stand-alone religious and spiritual interventions and how these methods can benefit older adults with depression. Because so many older adults express a preference for including religion and spirituality in treatment and because of the preliminary promising results of several studies, this is an area of research that should not be overlooked. Finally, because older adults have to cope with end of life issues, these therapies may be especially well suited for this issue and deserve further research in this aspect.

SUMMARY

The use of CAM for treatment of depression in older people is a promising area of psychiatry that deserves further study. The interventions reviewed in this article are noted for their mostly benign nature, the relative ease for combining with standard therapies (although caution needs to be taken with natural remedies), relative accessibility, and ease of implementation. The delivery of some of these interventions in a group format may also provide the added benefit of social interaction, which older people often lack.[138] Clinicians who are treating elderly patients with depression should consider these interventions carefully and discuss their pros and cons in detail before decisions are made as to whether a patient should seek them out.

CLINICAL VIGNETTE: **CAM** FOR **MAJOR DEPRESSIVE DISORDER**

History: *Mr K was a 70-year-old married white man with a history of mild but persistent MDD. The onset of his depression began at approximately age 60, after his oldest son died of cancer. Mr K's medical history was significant for mild hypertension, a result of being 15 to 20 pounds overweight most of his adult life. His hypertension was treated with β-blockers; although he tolerated them well, he often worried that they could exacerbate his depression. The patient tried several prescription antidepressants, with mild benefit, but generally required discontinuation due to side effects, in particular sexual dysfunction.*

New psychiatric evaluation: *Mr K met criteria for a major depressive episode, most notably poor sleep and fatigue. While obtaining Mr K's history, the psychiatrist inquired about use of over-the-counter supplements. Mr K denied use, although he expressed curiosity about natural antidepressants after recently seeing a report on a news show. His interest was due largely to their apparently benign side-effect profiles. Because the patient's depression was mild and he denied any suicidal ideation, the psychiatrist discussed 3 natural products, including omega-3 fatty acids, SAMe, and SJW. Mr K declined SJW due to concerns about interactions with his other medications and thought that SAMe would be too expensive to pay for out of pocket. He agreed to a trial of an EPA-DHA combination at 1000 mg/d.*

Outcome at 2 months: *Mr K reported mild improvement in mood and noted that his cardiologist had been pleased with some "unexplained" improvement in his serum lipid profiles. The cardiologist had also emphasized the need for weight loss, although Mr K was reluctant to take up a rigorous exercise program at his age. The psychiatrist suggested a yoga class for elderly people that a colleague of his attended. Mr K decided to sample a class and found that he liked it. He started practicing regularly (2× per week) while continuing the omega-3 supplement. After 6 months, his mood, sleep, and energy improved. He also lost 15 pounds, and his blood pressure normalized such that his cardiologist discontinued the β-blocker. Discontinuing the β-blocker also helped Mr K's mood, and he noted further improvement in his sexual function. At this time, Mr K continues his regimen of yoga and omega-3 and reports feeling as good as ever.*

REFERENCES

1. Bottino CM, Barcelos-Ferreira R, Ribeiz SR. Treatment of depression in older adults. Curr Psychiatry Rep 2012;14:289–97.
2. Wagenaar DB, Mickus MA, Gaumer KA, et al. Late-life depression and mental health services in primary care. J Geriatr Psychiatry Neurol 2002;15:134–40.
3. Eisenberg DM, Davis RB, Ettner SL, et al. Trends in alternative medicine use in the United States, 1990–1997: results of a follow-up national survey. JAMA 1998; 280:1569–75.
4. Barnes PM, Powell-Griner E, McFann K, et al. Complementary and alternative medicine use among adults: United States, 2002. Adv Data 2004;(343):1–19.
5. Flaherty JH, Takahashi R. The use of complementary and alternative medical therapies among older persons around the world. Clin Geriatr Med 2004;20: 179–200, v.
6. Mischoulon D. Update and critique of natural remedies as antidepressant treatments. Obstet Gynecol Clin North Am 2009;36:789–807.
7. Mischoulon D, Rosenbaum JF. Complementary and alternative medicine in society: an introduction. In: Mischoulon D, Rosenbaum J, editors. Natural medications for psychiatric disorders: considering the alternatives. 2nd edition. Philadelphia: Lippincott Williams & Wilkins; 2008. p. 3–10.
8. Lavretsky H. Complementary and alternative medicine use for treatment and prevention of late-life mood and cognitive disorders. Aging health 2009;5: 61–78.

9. Harrer G, Schmidt U, Kuhn U, et al. Comparison of equivalence between the St. John's wort extract LoHyp-57 and fluoxetine. Arzneimittelforschung 1999;49: 289–96.

10. Mannel M, Kuhn U, Schmidt U, et al. St. John's wort extract L160 for the treatment of depression with atypical features-a double-blind randomized, and placebo controlled trial. J Psychiatr Res 2010;44:760–7.

11. Dinamarca MC, Cerpa W, Garrido J, et al. Hyperforin prevents β-amyloid neurotoxicity and spatial memory impairments by disaggregation of Alzheimer's amyloid-β-deposits. Mol Psychiatry 2006;11:1032–48.

12. Freeman MP, Hibbeln JR, Wisner KL, et al. Omega-3 fatty acids: evidence basis for treatment and future research in psychiatry. J Clin Psychiatry 2006;67: 1954–67.

13. Sublette ME, Ellis SP, Geant AL, et al. Meta-analysis of the effects of eicosapentaenoic acid (EPA) in clinical trials in depression. J Clin Psychiatry 2011;72: 1577–84.

14. Bloch MH, Hannestad J. Omega-3 fatty acids for the treatment of depression: systematic review and meta-analysis. Mol Psychiatry 2012;17:1272–82.

15. Rondanelli M, Giacosa A, Opizzi A, et al. Effect of omega-3 fatty acids supplementation on depressive symptoms and on health-related quality of life in the treatment of elderly women with depression: a double-blind, placebo-controlled, randomized clinical trial. J Am Coll Nutr 2010;29:55–64.

16. Martins JG, Bentsen H, Puri BK. Eicosapentaenoic acid appears to be the key omega-3 fatty acid component associated with efficacy in major depressive disorder: a critique of Bloch and Hannestad and updated meta-analysis. Mol Psychiatry 2012;17:1144–9.

17. Lin PY, Mischoulon D, Freeman MP, et al. Are omega-3 fatty acids antidepressants or just mood-improving agents? The effect depends upon diagnosis, supplement preparation, and severity of depression. Mol Psychiatry 2012;17: 1161–3.

18. Bloch MH, Hannestad J. Response to critiques on 'Omega-3 fatty acids for the treatment of depression: systematic review and meta-analysis'. Mol Psychiatry 2012;17:1163–7.

19. Fotuhi M, Mohassel P, Yaffe K. Fish consumption, long-chain omega-3 fatty acids and risk of cognitive decline or Alzheimer disease: a complex association. Nat Clin Pract Neurol 2009;5:140–52.

20. Kremer JM, Lawrence DA, Petrillo GF, et al. Effects of high dose fish oil on rheumatoid arthritis after stopping nonsteroidal antiinflammatory drugs. Arthritis Rheum 1995;38:1107–14.

21. Mischoulon D, Fava M. Role of S-adenosyl-L-methionine in the treatment of depression: a review of the evidence. Am J Clin Nutr 2002;76(Suppl 5): 1158S–61S.

22. Papakostas GI. Evidence for S-adenosyl-L-methionine (SAM-e) for the treatment of major depressive disorder. J Clin Psychiatry 2009;70(Suppl 5):18–22.

23. Alvarez E, Udina C, Guillamat R. Shortening of latency period in depressed patients treated with SAMe and other antidepressant drugs. Cell Biol Rev 1987;S1:103–10.

24. Berlanga C, Ortega-Soto HA, Ontiveros M, et al. Efficacy of S-adenosyl-L-methionine in speeding the onset of action of imipramine. Psychiatry Res 1992;44: 257–62.

25. Alpert JE, Papakostas G, Mischoulon D, et al. S-Adenosyl-l-methionine (SAMe) as an adjunct for resistant major depressive disorder: an open trial following

partial or nonresponse to selective serotonin reuptake inhibitors or venlafaxine. J Clin Psychopharmacol 2004;24:661–4.

26. Papakostas GI, Mischoulon D, Shyu I, et al. S-adenosyl Methionine (SAMe) augmentation of serotonin reuptake inhibitors (SRIs) for SRI-non-responders with major depressive disorder: a double-blind, randomized clinical trial. Am J Psychiatry 2010;167:942–8.

27. Alpert JE, Papakostas GI, Mischoulon D. One-carbon metabolism and the treatment of depression: roles of s-adenosyl-l-methionine and folate. In: Mischoulon D, Rosenbaum J, editors. Natural medications for psychiatric disorders: considering the alternatives. 2nd edition. Philadelphia: Lippincott Williams & Wilkins; 2008. p. 68–83.

28. Fontanari D, DiPalma C, Giorgetti G, et al. Effects of S-adenosyl- L-methionine on cognitive and vigilance functions in elderly. Curr Ther Res 1994;55:682–9.

29. Di Rocco A, Rogers JD, Brown R, et al. S-Adenosyl-methionine improves depression in patients with Parkinson's disease in an open-label clinical trial. Mov Disord 2000;15:1225–9.

30. Mischoulon D, Raab MF. The role of folate in depression and dementia. J Clin Psychiatry 2007;68(Suppl 10):28–33.

31. Mischoulon D, Fava M, Stahl S. Folate supplementation [response to letter]. J Clin Psychiatry 2009;70:767–9.

32. Papakostas GI, Shelton RC, Zajecka JM, et al. l-Methylfolate as adjunctive therapy for SSRI-resistant major depression: results of two randomized, double-blind, parallel-sequential trials. Am J Psychiatry 2012;169:1267–74.

33. Larson EB, Bruce RA. Health benefits of exercise in an aging society. Arch Intern Med 1987;147:353–6.

34. Penedo FJ, Dahn JR. Exercise and well-being: a review of mental and physical health benefits associated with physical activity. Curr Opin Psychiatry 2005;18: 189–93.

35. Warburton DE, Nicol CW, Bredin SS. Health benefits of physical activity: the evidence. CMAJ 2006;174:801–9.

36. Strawbridge WJ, Deleger S, Roberts RE, et al. Physical activity reduces the risk of subsequent depression for older adults. Am J Epidemiol 2002;156: 328–34.

37. Blumenthal JA, Babyak MA, Moore KA, et al. Effects of exercise training on older patients with major depression. Arch Intern Med 1999;159:2349–56.

38. Blumenthal JA, Babyak MA, Doraiswamy PM, et al. Exercise and pharmacotherapy in the treatment of major depressive disorder. Psychosom Med 2007; 69:587–96.

39. Trivedi MH, Greer TL, Church TS, et al. Exercise as an augmentation treatment for nonremitted major depressive disorder: a randomized, parallel dose comparison. J Clin Psychiatry 2011;72:677–84.

40. Barbour KA, Blumenthal JA. Exercise training and depression in older adults. Neurobiol Aging 2005;26(Suppl 1):119–23.

41. Fukukawa Y, Nakashima C, Tsuboi S, et al. Age differences in the effect of physical activity on depressive symptoms. Psychol Aging 2004;19:346–51.

42. Babyak M, Blumenthal JA, Herman S, et al. Exercise treatment for major depression: maintenance of therapeutic benefit at 10 months. Psychosom Med 2000; 62:633–8.

43. Timonen L, Rantanen T, Timonen TE, et al. Effects of a group-based exercise program on the mood state of frail older women after discharge from hospital. Int J Geriatr Psychiatry 2002;17:1106–11.

44. Mather AS, Rodriguez C, Guthrie MF, et al. Effects of exercise on depressive symptoms in older adults with poorly responsive depressive disorder: randomised controlled trial. Br J Psychiatry 2002;180:411–5.
45. Sjösten N, Kivelä SL. The effects of physical exercise on depressive symptoms among the aged: a systematic review. Int J Geriatr Psychiatry 2006; 21:410–8.
46. Singh NA, Clements KM, Fiatarone MA. A randomized controlled trial of progressive resistance training in depressed elders. J Gerontol A Biol Sci Med Sci 1997;52A:M27–35.
47. McNeil JK, LeBlanc EM, Joyner M. The effect of exercise on depressive symptoms in the moderately depressed elderly. Psychol Aging 1991;6:487–8.
48. Dunn AL, Andersen RE, Jakicic JM. Lifestyle physical activity interventions. History, short- and long-term effects, and recommendations. Am J Prev Med 1998; 15:398–412.
49. Kodis J, Smith KM, Arthur HM, et al. Changes in exercise capacity and lipids after clinic versus home-based aerobic training in coronary artery bypass graft surgery patients. J Cardiopulm Rehabil 2001;21:31–6.
50. Dunn AL, Trivedi MH, Kampert JB, et al. Exercise treatment for depression: efficacy and dose response. Am J Prev Med 2005;28:1–8.
51. Ströhle A. Physical activity, exercise, depression and anxiety disorders. J Neural Transm 2009;116:777–84.
52. Martinsen EW. Physical activity and depression: clinical experience. Acta Psychiatr Scand Suppl 1994;377:23–7.
53. Arent SM, Landers DM, Etnier JL. The effects of exercise on mood in older adults: a meta-analytic review. J Aging Phys Activ 2000;8:407–30.
54. Ransford CP. A role for amines in the antidepressant effect of exercise: a review. Med Sci Sports Exerc 1982;14:1–10.
55. Sothmann MS, Ismail AH. Relationships between urinary catecholamine metabolites, particularly MHPG, and selected personality and physical fitness characteristics in normal subjects. Psychosom Med 1984;46:523–33.
56. Dishman RK. Brain monoamines, exercise, and behavioral stress: animal models. Med Sci Sports Exerc 1997;29:63–74.
57. Cho HJ, Lavretsky H, Olmstead R, et al. Sleep disturbance and depression recurrence in community-dwelling older adults: a prospective study. Am J Psychiatry 2008;165:1543–50.
58. Sherman KJ. Guidelines for developing yoga interventions for randomized trials. Evid Based Complement Alternat Med 2012;2012:143271.
59. Birdee GS, Legedza AT, Saper RB, et al. Characteristics of yoga users: results of a national survey. J Gen Intern Med 2008;23:1653–8.
60. Sengupta P. Health impacts of yoga and pranayama: a state-of-the-art review. Int J Prev Med 2012;3:444–58.
61. Evans S, Moieni M, Lung K, et al. Impact of iyengar yoga on quality of life in young women with rheumatoid arthritis. Clin J Pain 2013. [Epub ahead of print].
62. Lakkireddy D, Atkins D, Pillarisetti J, et al. Effect of yoga on arrhythmia burden, anxiety, depression, and quality of life in paroxysmal atrial fibrillation: the YOGA my heart study. J Am Coll Cardiol 2013;61(11):1177–82 pii:S0735-1097(13) 00044-2.
63. Cramer H, Lauche R, Hohmann C, et al. Randomized-controlled trial comparing yoga and home-based exercise for chronic neck pain. Clin J Pain 2013;29: 216–23.

64. Bidwell AJ, Yazel B, Davin D, et al. Yoga training improves quality of life in women with asthma. J Altern Complement Med 2012;18:749–55.
65. Buffart LM, van Uffelen JG, Riphagen II, et al. Physical and psychosocial benefits of yoga in cancer patients and survivors, a systematic review and meta-analysis of randomized controlled trials. BMC Cancer 2012;12:559.
66. Bussing A, Ostermann T, Ludtke R, et al. Effets of yoga interventions on pain and pain-associated disability: a meta-analysis. J Pain 2012;13:1–9.
67. Michalsen A, Jeitler M, Brunnhuber S, et al. Iyengar yoga for distressed women: a 3-armed randomized controlled trial. Evid Based Complement Alternat Med 2012;2012:408727.
68. Patel NK, Newstead AH, Ferrer RL. The effects of yoga on physical functioning and health related quality of life in older adults: a systematic review and meta-analysis. J Altern Complement Med 2012;18:902–17.
69. Alexander GK, Innes KE, Selfe TK, et al. "More than I expected": perceived benefits of yoga practice among older adults at risk for cardiovascular disease. Complement Ther Med 2013;21:14–28.
70. Uebelacker LA, Epstein-Lubow G, Gaudiano BA, et al. Hatha yoga for depression: critical review of the evidence for efficacy, plausible mechanisms of action, and directions for future research. J Psychiatr Pract 2010;16:22–33.
71. Balasubramaniam M, Telles S, Doraiswamy PM. Yoga on our minds: a systematic review of yoga for neuropsychiatric disorders. Front Psychiatry 2012;3:117.
72. Krishnamurthy MN, Telles S. Assessing depression following two ancient Indian interventions: effects of yoga and ayurveda on older adults in a residential home. J Gerontol Nurs 2007;33:17–23.
73. Bora E, Harrison BJ, Yucel M, et al. Cognitive impairment in euthymic major depressive disorder: a meta-analysis. Psychol Med 2013;43:2017–26.
74. Rocha KK, Ribeiro AM, Rocha KC, et al. Improvement in physiological and psychological parameters after 6 months of yoga practice. Conscious Cogn 2012; 21:843–50.
75. Oken BS, Zajdel D, Kishiyama S, et al. Randomized, controlled, six-month trial of yoga in healthy seniors: effects on cognition and quality of life. Altern Ther Health Med 2006;12:40–7.
76. Leuchter AF, Cook IA, Hamilton SP, et al. Biomarkers to predict antidepressant response. Curr Psychiatry Rep 2010;12:553–62.
77. Li AW, Goldsmith CA. The effects of yoga on anxiety and stress. Altern Med Rev 2012;17:21–35.
78. Satyapriya M, Nagendra HR, Nagarathna R, et al. Effect of integrated yoga on stress and heart rate variability in pregnant women. Int J Gynaecol Obstet 2009;104:218–22.
79. Sathyaprabha TN, Satishchandra P, Pradhan C, et al. Modulation of cardiac autonomic balance with adjuvant yoga therapy in patients with refractory epilepsy. Epilepsy Behav 2008;12:245–52.
80. Khattab K, Khattab AA, Ortak J, et al. Iyengar yoga increases cardiac parasympathetic nervous modulation among healthy yoga practitioners. Evid Based Complement Alternat Med 2007;4:511–7.
81. Vadiraja HS, Raghavendra RM, Nagarathna R, et al. Effects of a yoga program on cortisol rhythm and mood states in early breast cancer patients undergoing adjuvant radiotherapy: a randomized controlled trial. Integr Cancer Ther 2009;8:37–46.
82. Vedamurthachar A, Janakiramaiah N, Hegde JM, et al. Antidepressant efficacy and hormonal effects of sudarshana kriya yoga (SKY) in alcohol dependent individuals. J Affect Disord 2006;94:249–53.

83. Kiecolt-Glaser JK, Christian L, Preston H, et al. Stress, inflammation, and yoga practice. Psychosom Med 2010;72:113–21.

84. Yadav RK, Magan D, Mehta N, et al. Efficacy of a short-term yoga-based lifestyle intervention in reducing stress and inflammation: preliminary results. J Altern Complement Med 2012;18:662–7.

85. Gooneratne NS. Complementary and alternative medicine for sleep disturbances in older adults. Clin Geriatr Med 2008;24:121–38.

86. Wojtek CZ. National expert meeting on Qi Gong and Tai Chi consensus report. Urbana (IL): UIUC; 2005.

87. Barnes PM, Bloom B, Nahin R. Complementary and alternative medicine use among adults and children: United States, 2007. Natl Health Stat Report 2008;12:1–23.

88. Butler LD, Waelde LC, Hastings TA, et al. Meditation with yoga, group therapy with hypnosis, and psychoeducation for long-term depressed mood: a randomized pilot trial. J Clin Psychol 2008;64:806–20.

89. Lan C, Chen SY, Wong MK, et al. Tai chi training for patients with coronary heart disease. Med Sport Sci 2008;52:182–94.

90. Barrow DE, Bedford A, Ives G, et al. An evaluation of the effects of Tai Chi Chuan and Chi Kung training in patients with symptomatic heart failure: a randomized controlled pilot study. Postgrad Med J 2007;83:717–21.

91. Yeh GY, Wang C, Wayne PM, et al. The effect of tai chi exercise on blood pressure: a systematic review. Prev Cardiol 2008;11:82–9.

92. Lai JS, Lan C, Wong MK, et al. Two-year trends in cardiorespiratory function among older Tai Chi Chuan practitioners and sedentary subjects. J Am Geriatr Soc 1995;43:1222–7.

93. Wolf SL, Sattin RW, Kutner M, et al. Intense tai chi exercise training and fall occurrences in older, transitionally frail adults: a randomized, controlled trial. J Am Geriatr Soc 2003;51:1693–701.

94. Lan C, Lai JS, Chen SY, et al. Tai Chi Chuan to improve muscular strength and endurance in elderly individuals: a pilot study. Arch Phys Med Rehabil 2000;81: 604–7.

95. Husted C, Pham L, Hekking A, et al. Improving quality of life for people with chronic conditions: the example of T'ai Chi and multiple sclerosis. Altern Ther Health Med 1999;5:70–4.

96. Wang C, Roubenoff R, Lau J, et al. Effect of Tai Chi in adults with rheumatoid arthritis. Rheumatology 2005;44:685–7.

97. Hartman CA, Manos TM, Winter C, et al. Effects of T'ai chi training on function and quality of life indicators in older adults with osteoarthritis. J Am Geriatr Soc 2000;48:1553–9.

98. Wang JS, Lan C, Wong MK. Tai Chi Chuan training to enhance microcirculatory function in healthy elderly men. Arch Phys Med Rehabil 2001;82:1176–80.

99. Irwin MR, Olmstead R, Oxman MN. Augmenting immune responses to varicella zoster virus in older adults: a randomized, controlled trial of Tai Chi. J Am Geriatr Soc 2007;55:511–7.

100. Wu G. Evaluation of the effectiveness of Tai Chi for improving balance and preventing falls in the older population–a review. J Am Geriatr Soc 2002;50:746–54.

101. Wayne P, Krebs D, Wolf S, et al. Can Tai Chi improve vestibulopathic postural control? Arch Phys Med Rehabil 2004;85:142–52.

102. Wayne PM, Kiel DP, Krebs DE, et al. The effects of Tai Chi on bone mineral density in postmenopausal women: a systematic review. Arch Phys Med Rehabil 2007;88:673–80.

103. Tsang HW, Chan EP, Cheung WM. Effects of mindful and non mindful exercises on people with depression: a systematic review. Br J Clin Psychol 2008;47: 303–22.

104. Wang C, Bannuru R, Ramel J, et al. Tai Chi on psychological well-being: systematic review and meta-analysis. BMC Complement Altern Med 2010;10:23.

105. Yeung A, Lepoutre V, Wayne P, et al. Tai Chi treatment for depressed Chinese Americans: a pilot study. Am J Phys Med Rehabil 2012;91:863–70.

106. Chou KL, Lee PW, Yu EC, et al. Effect of Tai Chi on depressive symptoms amongst Chinese older patients with depressive disorders: a randomized clinical trial. Int J Geriatr Psychiatry 2004;19:1105–7.

107. Lavretsky H, Alstein LL, Olmstead RE, et al. Complementary use of Tai Chi chih augments escitalopram treatment of geriatric depression: a randomized controlled trial. Am J Geriatr Psychiatry 2011;19:839–50.

108. Benson H, Beary JF, Carol MP. The relaxation response. Psychiatry 1974;37: 37–46.

109. Wallace KR, Benson H, Wilson AF. A wakeful hypometabolic physiologic state. Am J Physiol 1971;221:795–9.

110. Yehuda R, Giller EL, Southwick SM, et al. Hypothalamic-pituitary-adrenal dysfunction in posttraumatic stress disorder. Biol Psychiatry 1991;30:1031–48.

111. Swaab DF, Bao AM, Lucassen PJ. The stress system in the human brain in depression and neurodegeneration. Ageing Res Rev 2005;4:141–94.

112. Abelson JL, Khan S, Liberzon I, et al. HPA axis activity in patients with panic disorder: review and synthesis of four studies. Depress Anxiety 2007;24:66–76.

113. Murphy M, Donovan S, Taylor E. The physical and psychological effects of meditation: a review of contemporary research with a comprehensive bibliography. 2nd edition. Petaluma (CA): Institute of Noetic Sciences; 1997.

114. Baer R. Mindfulness training as a clinical intervention: a conceptual and empirical review. Clin Psychol Sci Pract 2003;10:125–43.

115. Walsh R, Shapiro SL. The meeting of meditative disciplines and Western Psychology: a mutually enriching dialogue. Am Psychol 2006;61:227–39.

116. Yeung A, Feldman G, Fava M. Self-management of depression: a manual for mental health and primary care professionals. Cambridge, UK: Cambridge University Press; 2010.

117. Hirakawa Y, Masuda Y, Kimata T, et al. Effects of home massage rehabilitation therapy for the bed-ridden elderly: a pilot trial with a three-month follow-up. Clin Rehabil 2005;19:20–7.

118. Sharpe PA, Williams HG, Granner ML, et al. A randomised study of the effects of massage therapy compared with guided relaxation on well-being and stress perception among older adults. Complement Ther Med 2007;15:157–63.

119. Cambron JA, Dexheimer J, Coe P, et al. Side-effects of massage therapy: a cross-sectional study of 100 clients. J Altern Complement Med 2007;13:793–6.

120. Bruscia KE. Standards of integrity for qualitative music therapy research. J Music Ther 1998;35:176–200.

121. Hadsell N. A sociological theory and approach to music therapy with adult psychiatric patients. J Music Ther 1974;11:113–24.

122. Benenzon R. Music therapy manual. Springfield, IL: Charles C. Thomas; 1981.

123. Chan MF, Chan EA, Mok E, et al. Effect of music on depression levels and physiological responses in community-based older adults. Int J Ment Health Nurs 2009;18:285–94.

124. Hanser SB, Thompson LW. Effects of a music therapy strategy on depressed older adults. J Gerontol 1994;49:P265–9.

125. Zerhusen J, Boyle K, Wilson W. Out of the darkness: group cognitive therapy for depressed elderly. J Psychosoc Nurs Ment Health Serv 1995;1:28–32.
126. Maratos AS, Gold C, Wang X, et al. Music therapy for depression. Cochrane Database Syst Rev 2008;(1):CD004517.
127. Chen X. Active music therapy for senile depression. Zhonghua Shen Jing Jing Shen Ke Za Zhi 1992;25:208–10, 252–3.
128. Maratos A, Crawford MJ, Procter S. Music therapy for depression: it seems to work, but how? Br J Psychiatry 2011;199:92–3.
129. Stanley MA, Bush AL, Camp ME, et al. Older adults' preferences for religion/ spirituality in treatment for anxiety and depression. Aging Ment Health 2011; 15:334–43.
130. Skarupski KA, Fitchett G, Evans DA, et al. Daily spiritual experiences in a biracial, community-based population of older adults. Aging Ment Health 2010;14: 779–89.
131. Rajagopal D, MacKenzie E, Bailey C, et al. The effectiveness of a spiritually-based intervention to alleviate subsyndromal anxiety and minor depression among older adults. J Relig Health 2002;41:153–66.
132. Moritz S, Quan H, Rickhi B, et al. A home study-based spirituality education program decreases emotional distress and increases quality of life–a randomized, controlled trial. Altern Ther Health Med 2006;12:26–35.
133. Phillips LL, Paukert AL, Stanley MA, et al. Incorporating religion and spirituality to improve care for anxiety and depression in older adults. Geriatrics 2009;64: 15–8.
134. Weisman de Mamani A, Tuchman N, Duarte E. Incorporating religion/spirituality into treatment for serious mental illness. Cognit Behav Pract 2010;17:348–57.
135. Hook JN, Worthington EL Jr, Davis DE, et al. Empirically supported religious and spiritual therapies. J Clin Psychol 2010;66:46–72.
136. Propst LR, Ostrom R, Watkins P, et al. Comparative efficacy of religious and nonreligious cognitive-behavioral therapy for the treatment of clinical depression in religious individuals. J Consult Clin Psychol 1992;60:94–103.
137. Rossiter-Thornton JF. Prayer in psychotherapy. Altern Ther Health Med 2000;6: 128, 125–7.
138. Nicholson NR. A review of social isolation: an important but underassessed condition in older adults. J Prim Prev 2012;33:137–52.

What Is the Role of Medications in Late Life Depression?

Rob M. Kok, MD, PhD

KEYWORDS

- Antidepressant • Treatment • Efficacy • Side effects

KEY POINTS

- Undertreatment of depression in the elderly is widespread.
- Antidepressants are as effective in the elderly as in younger adults if an adequate dose is used, and the elderly may require dosages used in younger adults.
- Antidepressants should be considered in patients with more severe depression and in patients with a mild to moderate depression who were unsuccessfully treated with non-pharmacological treatment.
- Evidence for a slower treatment response in the elderly compared with younger adults is sparse and contradictory.
- Pharmacologic treatment should never be the only treatment that a depressed older patient receives, but should be combined with psychological modalities and social interventions.

INTRODUCTION

The indication for pharmacologic treatment of depression in the elderly does not differ much from younger adults. However, undertreatment of depression in the elderly is widespread,[1] probably because of different factors including doubts about the efficacy and fear of adverse effects. In this article, we will discuss whether more recent data from randomized controlled trails (RCTs) and meta-analyses support these widely held beliefs, derived primarily from clinical observations of older inpatients 3 decades ago.

Pharmacologic treatment should never be the only treatment that a depressed older patients receives, but should be combined with psychological modalities (at least psycho-education, and if indicated, also psychotherapy) and social interventions. Data from studies where different treatment modalities were compared are scant,

Disclosure: The author has received research grants from Wyeth and Lundbeck and speaker's honoraria from GlaxoSmithKline, Lundbeck, Pfizer, and Wyeth.
Department of Old Age Psychiatry, Parnassia Psychiatric Institute, Mangostraat 1, The Hague 2552 KS, The Netherlands
E-mail address: r.kok@parnassia.nl

Psychiatr Clin N Am 36 (2013) 597–605
http://dx.doi.org/10.1016/j.psc.2013.08.006
0193-953X/13/$ – see front matter © 2013 Elsevier Inc. All rights reserved.

Abbreviations: Role of Medications in Late Life Depression	
CI	Confidence interval
ECT	Electroconvulsive therapy
NNT	Numbers-needed-to-treat
RCT	Randomized controlled trial
SSRI	Selective serotonin reuptake inhibitor
TCA	Tricyclic antidepressant

and the critical question, which depressed patients should be treated with what kind of treatment, cannot be answered based on studies in the elderly. Most guidelines however suggest that more severe depression may better be treated with antidepressants (or ECT), but some reviews also suggest that even more severe depression in the elderly may be treated with psychotherapy.[2] In addition, patients with a mild to moderate depression who were unsuccessfully treated with psychological treatment or, in a stepped care approach, have been treated unsuccessfully with, for example, physical exercise or a *coping with depression* course (see Francis and Kumar and Nyer, Doorley, Durham, and colleagues in this issue) should also be considered for treatment with antidepressants. Some elderly patients may have a serious medical illness that is a contraindication for the use of antidepressants, but this was more often the case in the older class of antidepressants (tricyclic antidepressants, TCAs). Many elderly depressed patients have a preference for psychological treatment, but the availability of trained psychotherapists is often limited.[3]

The aim of every treatment is to produce (and maintain) a remission rather than a response. Ratings scales are very helpful to ensure that this goal is achieved and should be used to monitor symptom reduction.

ANTIDEPRESSANTS

All different classes of antidepressants are used for the treatment of depression in the elderly. Antidepressant class has a strong relationship with adverse effects, and to a much lesser degree with efficacy. Selective serotonin reuptake inhibitors (SSRIs) are the most prescribed class of antidepressants and many guidelines advise these as first-line treatment in the elderly, as in younger adults.

Older patients frequently bear a high burden of medical illnesses and are often subject to the use of multiple medications, which may result in drug-drug interactions. Age-related pharmacokinetic changes may result in a wider range of drug concentrations in the elderly and pharmacodynamic changes make elderly patients more sensitive to side effects of antidepressants,[4] which means that in case of lithium or TCAs where reference values are known, a serum level is essential to establish the optimum dose of these drugs in the elderly. Another consequence is that general dosing guidelines, as for example that elderly need one-third to one-half of the adult dose, will result in too low doses in some cases and too high doses in other cases. There are insufficient data to establish the minimally effective dose for the SSRIs and other antidepressants, but most RCTs allowed a wider range, but not necessary a lower dose, in the elderly compared with younger adults. Whether this is also true in the very elderly, who are typically underrepresented in RCTs in the elderly, is not clear. Many textbooks advise in the elderly a *start low, go slow* approach, to minimize adverse effects. However, evidence is scant to support this view in the use of TCAs and has never been tested in the case of SSRIs and other antidepressants. The author suggests that *start low, then go and go all the way* may be a better advice in the elderly. In the author's experience, if a patient has no or minimum adverse effects in the first few days after an antidepressant is started, the dose can be increased every 2 to 4 days. A slower dose escalation schedule may be responsible for the longer time to achieve a remission that was found in a few studies in the elderly. Overall, the evidence for a slower response to antidepressants is sparse and contradictory.[5] Extending a trial over 8 weeks probably only benefits patients who have demonstrated at least a partial response (for example, at least 25% reduction on a depression rating scale) in the first 4 to 6 weeks after the start of an antidepressant.

EFFICACY OF ANTIDEPRESSANTS

Only 25 years ago, one of the first reviews of the efficacy of antidepressants in depression in the older patients found only 12 double-blind RCTs.[6] A more recent review found more than 100 RCTs in depressed patients without dementia.[7] Many reviews and meta-analyses have been published, and all placebo-controlled studies concluded that antidepressants are superior to placebo.[7-14] Few reviews directly compare efficacy of antidepressants in different age groups and conclude that older patients were just as likely as younger patients to go into remission after treatment.[15] However, all meta-analyses that calculated response or remission rates in elderly concluded that this did not differ from these rates in younger adults. In addition, within the group of elderly patients, no difference was found in antidepressant response between "young-old" (aged 59–69), "middle-old" (70–75), and "old-old" (76–99) subjects.[16] In the most recent of these meta-analyses, a response rate of 48% and a remission rate of 33.7% were found, both very similar to response and remission rates found in adult patients,[7] which means that there is no evidence base for the longstanding clinical belief that the efficacy of treatment of elderly depressed patients is lower compared with younger adults. Although age may not have an effect on treatment response, the age-associated increase in medical burden is often associated with a lower treatment response. However, a recent review of depression in adult patients with depression and chronic physical health problems included 63 placebo-controlled RCTs and found that both SSRIs and TCAs were superior to placebo.[17] Unfortunately, most RCTs in the elderly exclude patients with serious or unstable medical conditions.[12]

Most of the reviews did not find a difference between classes of antidepressants in older patients, including a more recent review specifically aimed at comparing single-action versus dual-action antidepressants.[18] One review found a smaller numbers-needed-to-treat (NNT) in the placebo controlled RCTs with TCAs (NNT 3.97, 95% confidence interval [CI] = 3.88–4.05) than with SSRIs (8.45; 95% CI = 8.38–8.53).[11] However, in studies directly comparing TCAs with SSRIs, no differences in efficacy were found. Unfortunately, many of these trials have been supported by a pharmaceutical company and did not use an optimal TCA treatment with the use of plasma level measurement.

In the author's review, they were also not able to replicate Anderson's finding regarding a better efficacy of TCAs among inpatients,[19] because there are not enough studies in older patients using the same outcome criteria to compare TCAs with SSRIs among only psychiatric inpatients.[7] Too few studies had included more severely depressed patients and therefore a replication of the important finding that antidepressants only separate from placebo in more severely ill patients, as suggested in a review of all trials submitted to the Food and Drug Administration for the licensing of 4 new generation antidepressants, was also not possible.[20]

There is no agreement which SSRI should be the first choice for the elderly. The side-effect profile of all SSRIs is equivalent and the differences in drug-drug interactions have only a limited clinical value as many of the interactions are with drugs that are not often prescribed anymore. Nortriptyline is a secondary amine that has been shown to induce less orthostatic hypotension than tertiary amines (eg, amitriptyline) and is the TCA of choice to treat depression in the elderly.

The treatment of depression in dementia patients is complicated, for example, by ethical issues in cases of noncompetence. Efficacy is not well established and demented patients are prone to more side effects. An earlier Cochrane review could include only 3 efficacy studies in the meta-analysis and concluded that the available evidence offered weak support to the contention that antidepressants are an effective treatment for patients with depression and dementia.[21] A more recent review found 7 trials with 330 participants.[22] The odds ratio for 6 trials reporting response rates with antidepressant and placebo was 2.12 (95% CI = 0.95–4.70; P = .07) and the odds ratio for 5 trials reporting remission rates was 1.97 (95% CI = 0.85–4.55; P = .11). The authors conclude that the evidence for antidepressant treatment of people with depression and dementia is suggestive but does not confirm efficacy, which is in line with the negative results from the largest published RCT to date, where treatment with sertraline or mirtazapine showed no significant difference in depression reduction after 3 months compared with the placebo group.[23] Interestingly, the lack of a statistically significant difference between antidepressants and placebo is in part due to a high placebo response, which is also found in other neuropsychiatric symptoms in dementia. This lack of a statistically significant difference may reflect a suboptimal level of usual care in many nursing homes, where many of these studies were conducted. Most reviews and guidelines agree that antidepressants should only be initiated in patients with a severe depression, or after an initial nonpharmacological strategy has failed.[24]

There is a paucity of double-blind RCTs in severely depressed patients, treatment-resistant depression, psychotic depression, minor depression, and depressed nursing home patients.[7]

SIDE EFFECTS OF ANTIDEPRESSANTS

Side effects are often not detected, and perhaps more importantly, many complaints from age-related physiologic changes or comorbid medical disorders may be attributed to the antidepressant with nonadherence as a result. To prevent both errors, a checklist with the most frequent side effects may be helpful before the start of the drug therapy.

Meta-analyses comparing the side effects of TCAs and SSRIs are contradictory. Mittmann and colleagues[8] could not demonstrate a statistically difference in safety (any side effect) between SSRIs and TCAs in an older study, but a more recent meta-analysis including 37 RCTs found that elderly recipients of TCAs had an increased withdrawal rate compared with SSRI recipients, and also specifically because of adverse effects.[25]

The use of TCAs has been limited since SSRIs and other antidepressant have become available with a better safety profile. The major safety issue of TCAs is their cardiovascular effect, resulting in an increased risk of sudden cardiovascular death in patients with ischemic heart disease, and a high mortality rate in healthy elderly after an overdose. The anticholinergic adverse effects of TCAs may also be problematic in the elderly, including dry mouth, urinary retention, and cognitive deterioration. TCAs are therefore not recommended as the first choice of treatment of depression in elderly patients. If orthostatic hypotension emerges, the risk of falls and other serious consequences must be balanced against the effectiveness of alternative treatments, but if there is a reason to continue the antidepressant, several treatments for orthostatic hypotension have been proven effective.[26]

In contrast, the use of SSRIs in the elderly does not seem to differ much from younger patients, with nausea, diarrhea, anorexia, headache, agitation, insomnia, sexual dysfunction, and hemorrhages as the most prominent side effects. The cardiovascular profile is relatively benign and these drugs are relatively safe in overdosage.[5] Other antidepressants, like mianserine, moclobemide, trazodone, venlafaxine, mirtazapine, bupropion, duloxetine, and agometaline, are a very heterogeneous group and have very different side-effects profiles.

TREATMENT RESISTANCE

About two-thirds of patients do not achieve remission in a single antidepressant trial.[7] If these patients are treated with a sequential treatment strategy, the vast majority of even severely depressed inpatients will finally achieve remission.[27] A recent systematic review of treatment of refractory depression in the elderly, defined as failure to respond to at least one course of treatment, found no double-blind placebo-controlled RCT in the elderly.[28] The overall response rate was 52% (95% CI 42–62), which is not different from the response rate of 48% found in nonrefractory patients.[7] Lithium augmentation was the best studied treatment option with a response rate of 42% (95% CI 21–65) and may be the first choice in cases of nonresponse.[29] Another effective treatment for treatment-resistant depression, electroconvulsive therapy, is discussed in McDonald, Riva-Posse, and Hermida in this issue.

MAINTENANCE

Once a remission is achieved, it is important to know how long the antidepressant should be continued. Only 8 double-blind RCTs with maintenance treatment in the elderly could be found, resulting in a reduction of 28% (95% CI: 21%–36%, $P<.00001$) of the risk of suffering a relapse or recurrence using antidepressants compared with placebo.[30] The NNT for the effect of continuation or maintenance treatment of all antidepressants is 3.6 (95% CI: 2.8–4.8). Recommendations for how long to continue the antidepressants cannot be made based on these RCTs alone. In a consensus guideline in older patients, most experts (56%) recommended continuing treatment for 1 year in single episodes. Less agreement was achieved in patients with 2 episodes whereby the most frequently endorsed advice (39%) was 2 years, but almost all experts (98%) recommended treatment for at least 3 years in older patients with 3 or more episodes.[31] In addition to the number of episodes, it is also suggested that the duration between the episodes and the severity should be taken into account.

MOOD STABILIZERS

The best evidence for mood stabilizers is in bipolar disorder, but in elderly patients the evidence is very limited and randomized studies are lacking. Lithium is the only mood stabilizer with an established efficacy in treatment-resistant depression (see above). Valproate is often used in elderly with a bipolar disorder, especially for acute mania or in mixed episodes, and also for preventing relapses. Based on anecdotal evidence and reviews of experts, the same serum levels as in adults are needed in the elderly.

The dose to reach this can vary greatly in the elderly, with some patients needing the same dose as in younger adults. Side effects are typically mild (sedation, weight gain, gastrointestinal effects) and relatively benign compared with other mood stabilizers, especially on cognitive function.[32]

Carbamazepine is used very infrequently in the elderly depressed unipolar patients, also in bipolar disorder, in a large part because of the unfavorable side-effect profile.

Lamotrigine is used more often in bipolar depression, but information in the elderly is, again, scarce. An open-label trial of lamotrigine augmentation in 57 older patients with either type I or type II bipolar depression, with a mean dose of 151 (SD 69) mg per day, found that lamotrigine was associated with improvement in depression, psychopathology, and functional status.[33]

PSYCHOSTIMULANTS

At present, psychostimulants have a very limited role in the treatment of depression.[34] These drugs have a history of use in depressed patients with medical illness, when there were contraindications to the use of TCAs and other drugs (for example, SSRIs) were not yet developed. Only one controlled RCT is published with elderly patients, in which methylphenidate was more effective than placebo in a small group of medical inpatients.[35] The major advantage of psychostimulants is their fast response, usually within 48 hours. Side effects are typically mild, especially changes in vital signs, and cardiac effects are uncommon. Controlled studies that compare psychostimulants with antidepressants are lacking.

NATUROPATHICS

Only one RCT is published on the efficacy of St John's Wort in the elderly, which was as effective as fluoxetine,[36] but patients were only mildly to moderately depressed. St John's Wort can cause drug-drug interactions because it can stimulate cytochrome P450, resulting in a lower level of other drugs.

A recent review of homeopathic treatments in psychiatry found no placebo-controlled studies of depression, neither in adults nor in the elderly.[37] Other alternative treatments are discussed in Nyer, Doorley, Durham, and colleagues in this issue.

SUMMARY

Antidepressants are as effective in the treatment of late-life depression as in younger patients. All antidepressants are equally effective in the elderly, if an adequate dose is used. Elderly are a heterogeneous group requiring an individualized approach to dosing, with many elderly needing the same dose as younger adults, especially with the newer antidepressants.

Antidepressants differ in their side-effects profile and the cardiovascular side effects of TCAs are the main reason that SSRIs (and sometimes also other antidepressants) are usually recommended as first choice of treatment of depression in elderly patients. Data from RCTs also suggest that older patients do not take longer to respond than younger patients.

Clinicians must realize that starting an antidepressant in the elderly means that potential adverse effects and even increased mortality due to comorbid physical illnesses should be balanced against the efficacy and side effects of alternative treatments, but that depression, if untreated, in itself has also a mortality risk.

A 78-year-old woman was referred to an outpatient clinic after a suicide attempt with 12 tablets of oxazepam 10 mg, combined with a moderate amount of alcohol. At first, she claimed that nothing was wrong with her, but later she admitted being depressed for more than a year. Two years ago her husband died, and in the first months after his death, she had many contacts with family and friends. When the visits gradually decreased, she became more and more depressed and started drinking wine every day, which she had never done before in her life. One year after the death of her husband, her daughter advised her to visit the general practitioner, who referred her to a bereavement support group. After a couple of sessions she felt somewhat better, but still suffered from depression and drank almost a bottle of wine each day.

At the time of admission, she presented with feelings of worthlessness, lack of concentration, anxiety, loss of appetite, early morning awakening, and fatigue. She refused psychotherapy, and citalopram 10 mg was started and after a few days increased to 20 mg/d. Side effects were moderate, but she was explained to that these would probably decrease after 1 to 2 weeks and she continued the medication. After 4 to 5 weeks she began to experience an improvement, and after 9 weeks she was feeling much improved. She had stopped drinking alcohol and was referred to a psychologist for bereavement therapy, because she still had many symptoms of mourning.

A 63-year-old man was admitted on an inpatient psychiatric ward a few weeks after being discharged from a general hospital where he had coronary artery bypass surgery after life-threatening angina pectoris. He has a long history of cardiovascular diseases (hypertension, heart failure, cardiac arrhythmias) and also suffers from obesity, diabetes mellitus, and macular degeneration with low vision. He has been depressed at least 4 times in the last 15 years, mostly after a serious medical condition but also after his early retirement. His wife explained that he always had difficulties coping with any changes in his life. After discharge of the general hospital, he was apathetic and refused a cardiac rehabilitation program. He did not want to live anymore, lost interest in his family, had strong feelings of guilt, was very tired, and lost his appetite. He also was convinced that the world was coming to an end and that this was his fault. He had used sertraline 100 mg/d for 5 years as maintenance treatment and the dose was increased to 200 mg/d. However, this did not improve his depression. A change to another SSRI for at least 6 weeks also did not improve his depression. Because there were no absolute contraindications to a TCA according to his cardiologist, nortriptyline was started at 25 mg and increased to 75 mg/d over 1 week. He had a serum level of 150 ng/mL with no serious changes on the EKG. However, even after 6 weeks no change at all was observed in his depression and augmentation with lithium was started and increased to a serum level of 0.92 mEq/L. Within 4 weeks he improved completely and started his cardiac rehab.

REFERENCES

1. Barry LC, Abou JJ, Simen AA, et al. Under-treatment of depression in older persons. J Affect Disord 2012;136:789–96.
2. Pinquart M, Duberstein PR, Lyness JM. Treatments for later-life depressive conditions: a meta-analytic comparison of pharmacotherapy and psychotherapy. Am J Psychiatry 2006;163:1493–501.
3. Gum AM, Arean PA, Hunkeler E, et al. Depression treatment preferences in older primary care patients. Gerontologist 2006;46:14–22.
4. Pollock BG. Pharmacokinetics and pharmacodynamics in late life. In: Roose SP, Sackeim HA, editors. Late-life depression. New York: Oxford University Press; 2004. p. 185–91.

5. Roose SP, Sackheim HA. Antidepressant medication for the treatment of late-life depression. In: Roose SP, Sackeim HA, editors. Late-life depression. New York: Oxford University Press; 2004. p. 192–202.

6. Gerson SC, Plotkin DA, Jarvik LF. Antidepressant drug studies, 1964 to 1986: empirical evidence for aging patients. J Clin Psychopharmacol 1988;8:311–22.

7. Kok RM, Heeren TJ, Nolen WA. Efficacy of treatment in older depressed patients: a systematic review and meta-analysis of double-blind randomized controlled trials with antidepressants. J Affect Disord 2012;141:103–15.

8. Mittmann N, Herrmann N, Einarson TR, et al. The efficacy, safety and tolerability of antidepressants in late life depression: a meta-analysis. J Affect Disord 1997; 46:191–217.

9. McCusker J, Cole M, Keller E, et al. Effectiveness of treatments of depression in older ambulatory patients. Arch Intern Med 1998;158:705–12.

10. Katona C, Livingston G. How well do antidepressants work in older people? A systematic review of number needed to treat. J Affect Disord 2002;69:47–52.

11. Wilson K, Mottram P, Sivanranthan A, et al. Antidepressant versus placebo for depressed elderly. Cochrane Database Syst Rev 2001;(1):CD000561.

12. Taylor WD, Doraiswamy PM. A systematic review of antidepressant placebo-controlled trials for geriatric depression: limitations of current data and directions for the future. Neuropsychopharmacology 2004;29:2285–99.

13. Nelson JC, Delucchi K, Schneider LS. Efficacy of second generation antidepressants in late-life depression: a meta-analysis of the evidence. Am J Geriatr Psychiatry 2008;16:558–67.

14. Sneed JR, Rutherford BR, Rindskopf D, et al. Design makes a difference; a meta-analysis of antidepressant response rates in placebo-controlled versus comparator trails in late-life depression. Am J Geriatr Psychiatry 2008;16:65–73.

15. Williams JW Jr, Mulrow CD, Chiquette E, et al. A systematic review of newer pharmacotherapy's for depression in adults: evidence report summary. Ann Intern Med 2000;132:743–56.

16. Gildengers AG, Houck PR, Mulsant BH, et al. Course and rate of antidepressant response in the very old. J Affect Disord 2002;69:177–84.

17. Taylor D, Meader N, Bird V, et al. Pharmacological interventions for people with depression and chronic physical health problems; systematic review and meta-analyses of safety and efficacy. Br J Psychiatry 2011;198:179–88.

18. Mukai Y, Tampi RR. Treatment of depression in the elderly: a review of the recent literature on the efficacy of single- versus dual-action antidepressants. Clin Ther 2009;31:945–61.

19. Anderson IM. Selective serotonin reuptake inhibitors versus tricyclic antidepressants: a meta-analysis of efficacy and tolerability. J Affect Disord 2000;58: 19–36.

20. Kirsch I, Deacon BJ, Huedo-Medina TB, et al. Initial severity and antidepressant benefits: a meta-analysis of data submitted to the Food and Drug Administration. PLoS Med 2008;5:e45.

21. Bains J, Birks JS, Dening TR. The efficacy of antidepressants in the treatment of depression in dementia. Cochrane Database Syst Rev 2002;(4):CD003944.

22. Nelson JC, Devanand DP. A systematic review and meta-analysis of placebo-controlled antidepressant studies in people with depression and dementia. J Am Geriatr Soc 2011;59:577–85.

23. Banerjee S, Hellier J, Dewey M, et al. Sertraline or mirtazapine for depression in dementia (HTA-SADD): a randomised, multicentre, double-blind, placebo-controlled trial. Lancet 2011;378:403–11.

24. Sink KM, Holden KF, Yaffe K. Pharmacological treatment of neuropsychiatric symptoms of dementia: a review of the evidence. JAMA 2005;293:596–608.
25. Wilson K, Mottram P. A comparison of side effects of selective serotonin reuptake inhibitors and tricyclic antidepressants in older depressed patients: a meta-analysis. Int J Geriatr Psychiatry 2004;19:754–62.
26. Logan IC, Witham MD. Efficacy of treatment for orthostatic hypotension: a systematic review. Age Ageing 2012;41:587–94.
27. Kok RM, Nolen WA, Heeren TJ. Outcome of late-life depression after 3 years of sequential treatment. Acta Psychiatr Scand 2009;119:274–81.
28. Cooper C, Katona C, Lyketsos K, et al. A systematic review of treatments for refractory depression in older people. Am J Psychiatry 2011;168:681–8.
29. Kok RM, Vink D, Heeren TJ, et al. Lithium augmentation compared with phenelzine in treatment-resistant depression in the elderly: an open, randomized, controlled trial. J Clin Psychiatry 2007;68:1177–85.
30. Kok RM, Heeren TJ, Nolen WA. Continuing treatment of depression in the elderly: a systematic review and meta-analysis of double-blinded randomized controlled trials with antidepressants. Am J Geriatr Psychiatry 2011;19:249–55.
31. Alexopoulos GS, Katz IR, Reynolds CF, et al. The expert consensus guideline series. Pharmacotherapy of depressive disorders in older patients. Postgrad Med 2001;1–86.
32. Bowden CL. Mood stabilizers. In: Roose SP, Sackeim HA, editors. Late-life depression. New York: Oxford University Press; 2004. p. 211–21.
33. Sajatovic M, Gildengers A, Al Jurdi RK, et al. Multisite, open-label, prospective trial of lamotrigine for geriatric bipolar depression: a preliminary report. Bipolar Disord 2011;13:294–302.
34. Nelson JC. Stimulants. In: Roose SP, Sackeim HA, editors. Late-life depression. New York: Oxford University Press; 2004. p. 222–31.
35. Wallace AE, Kofoed LL, West AN. Double-blind, placebo-controlled trial of methylphenidate in older, depressed, medically ill patients. Am J Psychiatry 1995;152:929–31.
36. Harrer G, Schmidt U, Kuhn U, et al. Comparison of equivalence between the St. John's Wort extract LoHyp-57 and fluoxetine. Arzneimittelforschung 1999; 49:289–96.
37. Davidson JR, Crawford C, Ives JA, et al. Homeopathic treatments in psychiatry: a systematic review of randomized placebo-controlled studies. J Clin Psychiatry 2011;72:795–805.

The Role of Electroconvulsive and Neuromodulation Therapies in the Treatment of Geriatric Depression

Patricio Riva-Posse, MD[a],*, Adriana P. Hermida, MD[a],
William M. McDonald, MD[b]

KEYWORDS

- Electroconvulsive therapy • Neuromodulation • Geriatric depression
- Treatment-resistant depression

KEY POINTS

- Somatic nonpharmacological interventions, with electroconvulsive therapy being the most evidence-based, safe, and validated by decades of clinical practice and research, are useful and essential options for treatment in the geriatric population with mood disorders.
- Newer approaches, most of them still experimental, are becoming more available, with significant differences in results, invasiveness, and side effect profiles.
- Focal neuromodulation strategies may become accessible tools in the next few years to use in the management of difficult-to-treat patients with severe mood disorders.
- Noninvasive strategies that do not require general anesthesia and are easily administered in the outpatient setting may be valuable adjuncts to the current treatment options.
- The most invasive methods, like deep brain stimulation, seem to offer encouraging results for those patients who have failed the first-line and second-line treatments.

INTRODUCTION

Geriatric depression is a public health problem associated with increased mortality because of suicide and decreases in functional and physical health.[1–4] In many elders, their depression is resistant to psychotherapy and medication and can become chronic.[1,2] These factors have led to the increasing use of electroconvulsive therapy (ECT) in the treatment of medication-resistant or life-threatening geriatric depression.

Multiple studies have supported the safety and efficacy of ECT in the elderly, even in patients older than 75 years with multiple medical comorbidities and cognitive

[a] Department of Psychiatry and Behavioral Sciences, Emory University, 101 Woodruff Cir NE, Suite 4000, Atlanta, GA 30322, USA; [b] Department of Psychiatry and Behavioral Sciences, Fuqua Center for Late-Life Depression, Emory University, 101 Woodruff Cir NE, Suite 4000, Atlanta, GA 30322, USA
* Corresponding author.
E-mail address: PRIVAPO@emory.edu

Psychiatr Clin N Am 36 (2013) 607–630
http://dx.doi.org/10.1016/j.psc.2013.08.007
0193-953X/13/$ – see front matter © 2013 Elsevier Inc. All rights reserved.

Abbreviations: Electroconvulsive and Neuromodulation Therapies in the Treatment of Geriatric Depression	
AD	Alzheimer disease
BF	Bifrontal
BPSD	Behavioral and psychological symptoms of dementia
BT	Bitemporal
CVA	Cerebrovascular accident
DBS	Deep brain stimulation
DLB	Dementia with Lewy bodies
DLPFC	Dorsolateral prefrontal cortex
ECT	Electroconvulsive therapy
FDA	Food and Drug Administration
FEAST	Focal electrically administered seizure therapy
MCI	Mild cognitive impairment
MST	Magnetic seizure therapy
PD	Parkinson disease
PIA	Postictal agitation
PSD	Poststroke depression
RUL	Right unilateral
tDCS	Transcranial direct current stimulation
rTMS	Repetitive transcranial magnetic stimulation
ST	Seizure threshold
TMS	Transcranial magnetic stimulation
VNS	Vagal nerve stimulation

impairment.[3,4] Yet, up to 20% of elderly patients may not respond to ECT, and the elderly are more susceptible to the cognitive side effects, including delirium and acute cardiovascular and other medical complications associated with ECT.

Improvements in ECT practice have focused on making the treatments safer and maintaining efficacy. One notable advance was the development of the brief pulse machines in the 1980s, and more recently, the refinement of the brief pulse to ultrabrief pulse treatment protocols. This technology allows the practitioner to deliver a more efficient stimulus dose, which decreases the stimulus charge and the cognitive side effects compared with the older sine wave machines.[5]

Another advance in technique focused on moving the electrodes away from the anatomic areas associated with verbal memory with the D'Elia right unilateral (RUL) placement[6] and later with bifrontal (BF)[7] and asymmetric electrode placements.[8] There was the recognition that the magnitude of the stimulus charge was associated with response and the stimulus dose could be limited to 1.5 to 2.5 times the seizure threshold (ST) for bitemporal (BT) ECT, which increased safety without any loss in efficacy.[9,10] All of these advances made ECT safer, with fewer cognitive side effects.

However, these advances did not necessarily improve the antidepressant response to ECT. BT ECT remains the gold standard, although there continue to be many older adults who have a partial or no response to BT ECT and others who have significant cognitive side effects. Alternative therapies are clearly needed for depressed geriatric patients who are resistant or intolerant to available somatic therapies.

Neuromodulation therapies may be important alternatives for the management of treatment-resistant depression in the elderly. Unlike ECT, the neuromodulation therapies are subconvulsive (eg, repetitive transcranial magnetic stimulation [rTMS] and transcranial direct current stimulation [tDCS]), focal (eg, magnetic seizure therapy [MST] and focal electrically administered seizure therapy [FEAST]) or subconvulsive and focal (eg, deep brain stimulation [DBS] and vagal nerve stimulation [VNS]). The potential of the neuromodulation therapies is that they can be focal and limit the stimulation of neuroanatomical structures associated with cognitive side effects. In addition, subconvulsive stimuli would also be less likely to affect cognition and be safer, because it would not require anesthesia. Therapies that combine both strategies could clearly be safer, but the question is whether they could be as effective as ECT. This review covers the available evidence on the safety and efficacy of ECT and the neuromodulation therapies in geriatric depression.

ECT

ECT is the most effective treatment in severely depressed elderly patients and can have manageable side effects, with transient adverse events and limited mortality using modern evidence-based protocols.[11,12] Depressed patients 65 years and older in community hospitals were 7 times more likely to receive ECT than patients aged 18 to 34 years.[13] Middle-aged and elderly patients have a higher remission rate after a course of ECT than younger patients,[3,13,14] remitted elderly after ECT have a lower relapse rate compared with younger patients,[15] and elderly individuals have more medical comorbidities, making them more vulnerable to side effects and drug-drug interaction from pharmacotherapy, higher rates of medication intolerance, and more frail presentations.[14] The depressed elderly also have increased disability and the associated risk of losing their independence if the depression is not adequately treated.[15] The efficacy of ECT in the elderly and the associated disability of severe treatment-resistant depression combine to make ECT an important modality for the depressed elderly.

Cardinal clinical features in the elderly with treatment-resistant depression have been shown to be particularly responsive to ECT. Suicidal ideation[16] and the risk of suicide[17] increase in the elderly, and ECT is effective in the rapid reduction of suicidal ideation.[18–20] Psychosis is also more common in late-life depression than depression in young adults and is also more likely to be resistant to medication.[21,22] Patients with symptoms of psychotic depression have been shown to have a higher remission rate and faster time to response than depressed patients without psychotic symptoms.[23,24]

Bipolar disorder accounts for 10% to 25% of all geriatric patients with mood disorders and 5% of all patients admitted to geropsychiatric inpatient units.[25] Bipolar disorder in the elderly is a disabling illness, frequently characterized by comorbid psychiatric disorders, including substance abuse, alcohol use disorders, dysthymia, generalized anxiety disorder, panic disorder,[26] and delirium.[27] ECT is an effective treatment of all phases of bipolar disorder,[25,28–46] although only a few studies have focused on elderly bipolar patients.[25,27,47–49]

ECT in Neuropsychiatric Disorders

Elderly patients referred to ECT for medication-resistant depression often present with comorbid neurodegenerative disorders, including mild cognitive impairment (MCI), dementia, Parkinson disease (PD), and stroke. ECT has been shown to be effective in treating mood disorders with comorbid neurological conditions and improving affective symptoms as well as agitation, motor deficits, and even cognition.

Parkinson disease

Major depression is a common nonmotor feature in PD, affecting approximately 40% of patients, with up to 94% presenting with subsyndromal depression.[50] Depression is more common in PD with prominent bradykinesia and gait instability than in tremor-dominant syndromes.[51] Nonmotor features significantly affect quality of life for both patients and their families and are a better predictor of distress than motor disability.[51]

ECT is beneficial in PD with comorbid depression[50,52] and parkinsonian motor symptoms that have not responded to typical treatments.[53] Motor symptoms have been shown to improve in PD independent of depressive symptoms,[54] and often, this improvement in motor symptoms preceded the improvement of depressive symptoms.[55] However, the benefits on motor symptoms are not permanent and may last only for a few days. Some have reported improvement lasting for several weeks or even up to 4 years with maintenance ECT.[56]

Careful consideration of electrode placement, frequency of treatment, and electrical charge administered should be taken when treating patients with PD with ECT. RUL ECT treatments twice per week, withholding the dose of levodopa on the morning of ECT, treating the patients with PD first thing in the morning, and holding ECT if delirium occurs are the general recommendations for ECT in PD.[57]

Alzheimer disease and other dementias

Depression is one of the most frequently diagnosed psychiatric disorders in patients with Alzheimer disease (AD) and other dementias. The prevalence of major and minor depression has been estimated to range between 30% and 50%; however, many cases are undiagnosed because symptoms of depression overlap dementia. Depression with comorbid dementia is responsive to ECT, although there is a higher risk of confusion and short-term memory loss.[58,59]

In addition to depression, there are other prominent behavioral symptoms in dementia, such as aggressive physical symptoms (throwing, grabbing, hitting, or kicking); aggressive verbal symptoms (swearing, cursing, or yelling); nonaggressive physical symptoms (pacing, repetitive inappropriate behaviors); and nonaggressive verbal symptoms (constant requests, chatting, and perseveration)[60–63]; defined as the behavioral and psychological symptoms of dementia (BPSD). BPSD are associated with increased functional impairment, premature institutionalization, increased mortality, and increased caregiver burden and total health care costs.[64]

The treatment of BPSD should be targeted to both environmental and pharmacological interventions, with emphasis on the use of nonpharmacological interventions. There is limited evidence supporting the efficacy of these interventions and no pharmacological interventions that have US Food and Drug Administration (FDA) approval for the treatment of BPSD. The role of ECT in the management of depression and BPSD in dementia is controversial, primarily because of the concern over worsening cognitive functioning and the difficulty in obtaining informed consent from the affected individual. However, there is an increasing body of literature about the use of ECT in the treatment of dementia with agitation and aggression, even in the absence of mood disorders.

Oudman[65] studied 19 patients with depression and dementia treated with ECT. The patients received a mean of 8.3 ECT treatments, with various electrode placements. Thirteen of the 19 patients showed improvements in depressive symptoms after ECT, and 9 had partial or full remission. Six patients had a worsening in general cognition, orientation, or memory, with improvement in the cognitive side effects over 10 to 65 days in 5 of the 6 patients. The same group reviewed 5 patients with multi-infarct dementia receiving ECT. The patients received a mean of 7.6 ECT treatments, and all improved significantly. However, 3 of the 6 patients experienced significant cognitive or memory improvement as a result of treatment with ECT, particularly when the patient who received BT ECT. Ujkaj and colleagues[66] retrospectively evaluated the efficacy and safety of ECT for agitation and aggression in demented patients who did not respond to behavioral and pharmacological treatments. These investigators concluded that ECT was both safe and effective for the treatment of agitation and aggression in dementia.

Dementia with Lewy bodies (DLB) has similar clinical features to PD (eg, cognitive problems including dementia, parkinsonian motor symptoms). DLB is the second most common dementing illness after AD in Western countries. The distinguishing clinical characteristic of PD with dementia and DLB is the timing of dementia onset.[67] Patients with DLB frequently present with depression, delusions, visual hallucinations, fluctuating cognition, and agitation. Estimates of depression associated with DLB range from 20% to 65%. Takahashi and colleagues[68] reported on 167 patients who were admitted to a psychiatric unit with mood disorders; 14% of these patients were subsequently diagnosed with DLB. Eight of these patients had a medication-resistant depression and received a course of 6 BT ECT. All of the 8 patients had a statistically significant reduction in their depressive symptoms, with no significant side effects. Rasmussen and colleagues[69] reported 7 patients with DLB, all with major depression and some with accompanying visual hallucinations or delusions, who received ECT with various electrode placements (RUL, BF, or BT). These investigators reported improvement in depressive symptoms in all 7 cases, with varying effects on visual hallucinations, delusions, and parkinsonian motor symptoms. The duration of the benefits ranged from 2 weeks to several months. Four of the 7 patients benefited from maintenance ECT, and the cognitive effects of ECT did not extend beyond the acute ECT period.

ECT should be considered in patients with dementia and severe, refractory behavioral symptoms.[64] Because ECT has antidepressant, antipsychotic, and dopamine-enhancing effects, it could address not only depressive symptoms but also psychosis and motor symptoms in patients with DLB, potentially avoiding a host of medication-related side effects.[66]

Cerebrovascular disease and stroke

The incidence of stroke increases with age[70]; each successive decade above 55 years has a doubling of stroke incidence.[71] Depression is the most common neuropsychiatric consequence of stroke. The risk of fatality is higher in patients with stroke with depression compared with nondepressed patients with stroke.[72] Depression is a significant clinical factor in at least one-third of patients in the first year after onset of stroke but could occur up to 2 to 3 years after stroke onset.[72] Recognition, assessment, and diagnosis of an underlying mood disorder associated with acute stroke are complex because of cognitive, language, and other sequelae from stroke.[73]

ECT is clinically indicated in patients with poststroke depression (PSD) who have significant depressive symptoms and have not responded to or tolerated antidepressant medication. However, there are no established guidelines on how long to wait after a stroke before ECT is administered to a patient with PSD with significant comorbid depression.

DeQuardo and Tandon[74] reported on a patient who had his first depressive episode as a complication of a right ischemic parietotemporal cerebrovascular accident (CVA) 15 months previously. The patient was treated with RUL ECT with excellent clinical results and without new neurological or neuropsychological deficits. In a retrospective chart review of 14 patients with PSD, Murray and colleagues[75] reported that 12 had a marked improvement in depression after a course of ECT. A transitory cardiac arrhythmia developed in 1 patient, but none of the patients had a worsening of their neurological status. These investigators concluded that ECT is safe and effective for PSD. Currier and colleagues[76] reviewed the medical records of 20 geriatric patients who received ECT for PSD. Of the 19 patients who improved with

ECT, 7 (37%) suffered relapses despite maintenance antidepressant medications. Five patients (23%) developed ECT-related medical complications. Three patients (15%) developed transient interictal confusion or amnesia. No patient experienced an exacerbation of preexisting neurological deficits, leading to the conclusion that ECT is generally a well-tolerated and effective treatment of depressed, medically ill poststroke geriatric patients. Weintraub and Lippmann[77] reported on a 79-year-old woman with a history of depression and an acute ischemic infarction in the left posterior inferior cerebellar artery, who responded to RUL ECT without observed complications. Harmandayan and colleagues[78] described a patient with a stroke sustained 6 months before ECT who responded successfully to ECT with no complications. Miller and Isenberg[79] described the case of a 58-year-old woman who developed aphasia, right-sided hemiparesis, and a possible right visual field defect after RUL ECT. The neurological deficits were reversible over a 3-day period.

Despite reports on the safety and efficacy of ECT in PSD, ECT after a CVA may worsen the neurological damage from the original stroke or may be associated with an increased incidence of delirium or cardiac complications. In addition, there are some reports of stroke during a course of ECT in vulnerable individuals. Bruce and colleagues[80] reported a case of ischemic stroke temporally related to ECT with radiological confirmation. Weisberg and colleagues[81] reported 1 patient who experienced intracerebral hemorrhage during a course of ECT.

ECT should be administered in the acute poststroke period only in settings in which adequate medical, neurological, and radiological consultations are available. Hemorrhagic strokes are associated with greater potential risks because of the possibility of rebleeding, so extra precautions have to be taken in this circumstance. Optimization of clotting factors, thorough medical evaluation, and close clinical monitoring of blood pressure are important measures for patient safety in patients with a higher risk of stroke.[82]

The Pre-ECT Workup in Geriatric Patients

An important consideration in the elderly is the consent process. Each US state (or each country in the European Union[83] or other counties) has their own laws regarding informed consent. These state-specific and country-specific laws should be considered in the consent process. However, the consent process in the elderly can be further complicated by the cognitive problems associated with depression in the elderly and because older patients may have specific challenges in the consent process, including an increased risk of dementia in geriatric depression.[84,85] Even considering these problems, the depressed elderly have been shown to have decisional capacity to consent to ECT and their capacity has increased significantly with education.[86] Providing educational materials in many different forms (eg, brochures, videos, active discussions with the doctor, involving family member) are particularly important in the informed consent process for older (and younger) patients.[87–89]

There are no absolute contraindications to ECT in the elderly, but the pretreatment medical assessment and anesthesia should be standardized and consider the high rate of medical comorbidities in this population. Although it was common practice 30 years ago for the psychiatrist to administer the ECT anesthesia often on the psychiatric unit, the present recommendations are for the pre-ECT evaluation and the ECT treatments to be under the supervision of a board-certified anesthesiologist in a medical suite suitable for general anesthesia.[90] The pretreatment medical evaluation should include a detailed history and physical examination as well as a review of all medications and the interval medical history before each treatment. The cardiac, pulmonary, and neurological examinations are the most important systems to focus on before starting ECT. Specialty consults should be considered in patients with unstable cardiac disease, focal neurological findings, and significant physical deconditioning, or poorly managed pulmonary disease. All patients older than 50 years should have baseline electrolytes, complete blood count, and 12-lead electrocardiography as well as any other laboratory examinations needed to assess their chronic medical conditions. Neuroimaging and radiological examinations (spine films or chest radiograph) are not necessarily part of the routine pre-ECT assessment but should be ordered when medically indicated.[90]

Anesthesia in Geriatric Patients

As noted earlier, older age is associated with increased STs and can result in missed seizures, particularly when administering suprathreshold RUL ECT in elderly males. Assuming that the anesthesiologist is using a combination of methohexital and succinylcholine, several strategies can be used to manage the ST, including adding an ultrashort-acting opioid and lowering the methohexital dose[91]; changing to etomidate as the anesthetic agent,[92] although this can cause post-ECT agitation; lowering the methohexital dose and adding ketamine[93]; adding flumazenil to patients on benzodiazepines[94]; sleep deprivation[95]; hyperventilation to obtain an end tidal volume CO_2 of at least 40 mm Hg with or without the use of a laryngeal airway mask[96]; or holding anticonvulsant medications.

Cardiovascular complications are rare but can be serious in the elderly,[97] and most of the complications are caused by known preexisting conditions.[98] To limit the cardiovascular complications, patients should take their prescribed cardiac medications on the morning before ECT and the anesthesiologist should administer cardiac medications immediately before the treatment as needed including β-blockers for tachycardia (eg, esmolol) and calcium channel blockers for hypertension (eg, nicardipine) or the combination of an α-blocker and β-blocker for both symptoms (eg, labetalol).[99–101]

Most cardiac pacemakers can be used safely during ECT, although there may be a small risk of ventricular tachycardia and fibrillation with asynchronous fixed-rate pacemakers, and special precautions are needed in patients with implantable cardioverter defibrillators.[102–104] Patients in atrial fibrillation can be treated safely but should undergo anticoagulation therapy before starting ECT.[105] Patients with abdominal aortic aneurysms and intracranial aneurysms have also been treated safely with ECT using modern evidence-based practices.[106–109]

Postictal agitation (PIA) can be a cause of injury for an elderly patient. Strategies to manage PIA include using propofol as the anesthetic agent. This agent is also associated with decreasing seizure durations compared with barbiturates.[110,111] Other strategies are to give midazolam or atypical antipsychotics immediately after the seizure. If a patient has significant PIA, our group has presented data showing that the use of dissolvable olanzapine (ie, Zydis) given immediately before the seizure is both safe and effective in preventing PIA after subsequent ECT treatments.[112]

Administering ECT in the Elderly

In elderly depressed patients who undergo a course of ECT, it is particularly important to maximize efficacy and minimize cognitive side effects. This balance is determined by the combination of electrode placement and electrical charge. Several modifications have been made to electrode placement to improve the cognitive profile of ECT, including moving the area of direct stimulation from the neuroanatomic areas most closely associated with memory (ie, BT ECT) to more direct cortical stimulation of the nondominant hemisphere (ie, RUL ECT) or frontal lobes (ie, BF ECT).[113,114]

Ultrabrief ECT technology
Advances in technology have led to a more efficient stimulus in depolarizing neurons and have therefore decreased the amount of energy needed to create a seizure. The replacement of the sine wave machines with brief pulse machines was a major development in ECT technology to improve the efficiency of the stimulus and decrease cognitive side effects.[115] Ultrabrief pulse technology (ie, pulse widths between 0.25 and 0.30 milliseconds) may allow practitioners to create seizures that are even more efficient and use less total energy,[116] with better cognitive outcomes.[117] Although the technology has been available for some time, caution should be noted in the use of ultrabrief ECT. Ultrabrief RUL has been shown to require more treatments than brief pulse RUL[117] and ultrabrief BT ECT was significantly less effective than either ultrabrief RUL or brief pulse RUL and brief pulse BT ECT in 1 study.[118] Another study[119] found that ultrabrief RUL had equivalent efficacy to ultrabrief BF ECT with good cognitive profiles for both treatments.

Seizure titration
Seizure titration refers to a technique that decreases the total amount of energy needed to generate a seizure. The ST is the amount of energy needed to create a seizure and is dependent on several variables, including increases with age and male gender.[120,121] Seizure titration is done in the first ECT session, and the practitioner gives gradually increasing amounts of energy until the patient has a generalized convulsion, which serves as the patient's ST. Titration is a method that individualizes the dosage of energy delivered to the individual's ST.

Once the ST has been established, the practitioner can determine the lowest effective dose of ECT as a starting point. Brief pulse RUL should be dosed supra-ST (6 times the ST), whereas BT ECT is effective at 1.5 to 2.5 the ST, and increasing higher than this dose increases cognitive side effects without increasing efficacy.[9,10,122] Given the data that antidepressant efficacy of RUL ECT is dependent on the magnitude of the stimulus dose relative to the ST, and a dose-response relationship extends to at least 12 times the ST,[122] increasing the dose in nonresponders after a set number of treatments is appropriate. However, the higher-dose RUL is also associated with increasing cognitive side effects whether the stimulus is brief pulse or ultrabrief pulse.[123]

These data all support ST in the elderly to maximize efficacy and minimize cognitive side effects. Some practitioners have described seizure titration as a troublesome and risky procedure.[124] Others have described safety concerns with ST, arguing that a subconvulsive stimulus carries the risk of unopposed vagal surge, which may elicit bradycardia, cardiac arrest, and other cardiovascular side effects.[125] A study by Prudic and colleagues[126] of the cognitive consequences of subconvulsive treatments in patients who underwent ECT and dose titration failed to show any additional cognitive adverse effects because of a subconvulsive stimulus.

Study comparing ECT dose titration with other dosing strategies
In a recent abstract presented by our group,[127] the dose titration method was compared with other dosing strategies such as half-age, age, and fixed-dose strategies within the 3 electrode placement modalities in 246 patients. We found that the age method resulted in overtreatment and possibly unnecessary cognitive side effects, whereas the half-age method and the fixed dose result in suboptimal treatment compared with the titration method. We had a predominantly geriatric population (76% were older than 55 years) and observed no cardiovascular events as a result of subconvulsive stimulus and all titrations were well tolerated.

The primary neurological complication during a course of ECT is delirium, which is less related to age and more to underlying neurological dysfunction, including atrophy, stroke, vascular disease including periventricular white matter disease, and chronic degenerative conditions, including PD and AD.[15,94,95] The subcortical hyperintensities that are found on the neuroimaging of patients diagnosed with vascular depression and older patients who are medication treatment resistant and referred to ECT are associated with a less than optimal response to ECT and an increase in delirium during ECT.[96–98,128]

Delirium monitoring

Monitoring elderly patients for subtle signs of delirium during an ECT course is important, because delirium can result in falls and PIA and may be the first sign of more significant long-term memory loss related to ECT. ECT-related delirium is often manifested as a hypoactive state, which can be difficult to distinguish from the psychomotor retardation noted in elderly patients with melancholic depression. A simple bedside test for interictal delirium is to ask the patient to recite the months backward, starting with December, and note the patient's speed and accuracy. This task is not education dependent and relies on the patient's attention, concentration, and psychomotor speed, which are the primary cognitive deficits in delirium.

Monitoring long-term and short-term memory can be more difficult. The most common tool used is the Mini-Mental State Examination,[129] which is insensitive to many of the cognitive changes that are associated with ECT. Depression is associated with cognitive complaints, particularly in the elderly. Some tasks may be more specific to depression (eg, acquisition of new information) and some tasks are more sensitive to the effects of ECT (eg, retention of learned information).[130] Subjective memory complaints are generally related to mood.[131] Anterograde memory usually recovers in the weeks after ECT but there can be long-term retrograde amnesia for general and autobiographical information.[5,132]

Generally, BT and BF ECT are associated with more persistent retrograde amnesia than RUL ECT[5,9,133]; however, when stimulus titration is used to dose BT and BF ECT at 1.5 times the ST and it is compared with RUL at 6 times the ST, all 3 electrode placements are safe and effective, with minimal long-term cognitive side effects.[134] The patients most at risk for more persistent retrograde amnesia are patients who are older, female, or have lower premorbid intellectual function[5] and those patients who manifest global cognitive impairment before ECT or who experience prolonged disorientation in the acute postictal period.[135] As noted earlier,[13] age alone does not increase the risk for ECT-related memory problems; rather, it is the association of age with cerebrovascular disease and neurological problems.

Strategies to manage cognitive problems include the use of brief pulse and ultrabrief RUL ECT, particularly in vulnerable groups of patients (eg, PD, AD),[117] administering ECT 2 times rather than 3 times a week[136] and various pharmacological strategies, including antidementia drugs (eg, donepezil, galantamine) in patients with preexisting cognitive impairment[59,137–140]; however, no 1 strategy has been found to be effective enough to gain general acceptance.

Maintenance ECT

Maintenance ECT is presently being evaluated in the National Institute of Mental Health–sponsored PRIDE (Preventing Relapse in Depressed Elderly) study. Although there are no published data yet from that study, the evidence for adults is a high relapse rate after ECT even in patients on maintenance medication[10] and maintenance ECT[141] (approximately 50%). Nevertheless, maintenance ECT is effective in the treatment of medication-resistant patients who remit from an index course of ECT,[142–147] particularly in combination with pharmacotherapy.[148,149] A 6-month course of maintenance ECT should be considered in patients who have relapsed on pharmacotherapy alone, and in many patients receiving maintenance ECT, the course may need to be extended beyond 6 months.[150] The most effective maintenance pharmacotherapy after ECT is a combination of lithium and nortriptyline,[151,152] although venlafaxine XR was as effective and is better tolerated in the elderly.[153] Lithium has also been associated with an increase in adverse events (eg, prolonged seizures, serotonin syndrome, delirium) in patients receiving ECT,[154–157] although some experts have questioned the safety of ECT and lithium therapy.[158,159] However, geriatric patients may not tolerate lithium, and alternative therapies should be considered, including monoamine oxidase inhibitors, atypical antipsychotic augmentation, and other novel treatments.

Summary of ECT

There is a rich dataset on the use of ECT in geriatric patients, including patients with neurodegenerative disease and comorbid medical problems. ECT is one of the safest procedures administered under general anesthesia, and these data guide modern ECT procedures. However, the number of elderly inpatients treated with ECT is declining largely because the number of hospitals providing ECT services has declined significantly.[61] This decline is hypothesized to be caused by the recent FDA review of the safety and efficacy of ECT and the review panel's recommendation to reclassify ECT devices into a more restrictive category.

The continued public misconceptions related to ECT and negative media depictions notwithstanding, the research community continues to provide compelling data on the safety and efficacy of ECT.[62,63] The elderly hold fewer misconceptions toward ECT than younger individuals.[64] Continued efforts are needed to develop and disseminate evidence-based protocols and improve the safety of the procedure.

NOVEL NEUROMODULATORY APPROACHES

Over the past 2 decades and with the development of advanced neuroimaging, depression is now widely viewed as a multidimensional, systems-level disorder affecting functionally integrated but discrete pathways.[160,161] This conceptualization has helped the growth of strategies that use focal neuromodulation to treat depression by directly affecting the activity of specific brain regions in order to modulate overall network function in a therapeutic way. These strategies include VNS, rTMS, DBS, tDCS, MST, and FEAST. The first 2 are FDA-approved, and the others are in different stages of development. These technologies are either subconvulsive or focal (if not both), hence avoiding the undesired cognitive side effects of ECT, the somatic nonpharmacological treatment with more evidence supporting its use. In the following sections, the evidence supporting its use as well as the experience in the geriatric population and the treatment of geriatric depression when available is reviewed.

VNS

VNS was approved by the FDA for use in chronic or recurrent depression in 2005. The observations of mood improvement in patients with treatment-resistant epilepsy receiving VNS therapy prompted its testing in patients with mood disorders. The improvement in depression was independent of the anticonvulsant efficacy.[162,163] Although its mechanism of action is not completely understood, there are several theories. Anticonvulsant agents are efficacious antidepressants and mood stabilizers.[164]

VNS has shown antidepressant activity in animal models of depression. It is believed to act through stimulation of the afferent fibers of the vagus nerve, which is closely linked with the mood-regulation networks, like the amygdala and brainstem structures (locus coeruleus).[165,166]

The VNS device consists of an implantable generator that is connected to electrodes that deliver low-frequency, chronic intermittent-pulsed electrical signals to the left cervical vagus nerve. Surgery is performed for implantation of a pacemakerlike programmable pulse generator device (NCP System, Cyberonics, Houston, TX). The generator is round, 50 mm (2 inches) in diameter, about 6.35 mm (one-quarter inch) thick, and weighs 25 g. It is implanted under general anesthesia as an outpatient procedure. Two incisions are made: the left upper chest or left axillary border (where the generator is implanted subcutaneously) and the left neck area (where the electrode lead wire is attached to the left vagus nerve). The lead wire is passed through a subcutaneous tunnel and attached to the pulse generator. Surgical complications can include wound infection (<2%) and hoarseness (because of temporary or permanent left vocal cord paralysis) in about 1% of patients.

Clinical response is slow but sustained. Response and remission rates have been lower than initially expected, and mostly shown by the long-term naturalistic follow-up of patients rather than in the primary, relatively short-term end points of the clinical trials.[167,168] The response and remission rates have been consistent around 28% and less than 10%, respectively.[168] One of the promising facts about VNS is the durability of the response, because sustained response rates at 2 years are reported to be between 53% and 78% of the initial responders to the stimulation.[169] Despite the approval by the FDA for clinical use, coverage by third-party payers has been limited.

In particular relevance to late-life depression and geriatric population, surgical complications have not been reported to be more frequent. In a VNS study of epilepsy in older patients, in whom the same procedure was performed, no cardiac abnormalities such as arrhythmias or asystole were reported during surgery.[170] It has also been reported to be a safe and well-tolerated procedure when used in a pilot study to treat patients with AD.[171]

Transcranial Magnetic Stimulation

Transcranial magnetic stimulation (TMS) is a noninvasive neuromodulatory technique approved by the FDA for the treatment of depression in adults who failed to respond to 1 medication trial. A potent relatively focal electromagnetic field is generated beneath a coil positioned over the scalp and it depolarizes neurons, modulating cortical activity. The most common stimulation parameter is performed at a high frequency (10 Hz) over the left dorsolateral prefrontal cortex (DLPFC), with sessions 5 times per week at 120% of motor threshold for 3000 pulses/session, during 4 to 6 weeks.[172] Slow-frequency TMS is also reported to have beneficial effects.[173] Potential benefits of rTMS over ECT include administration without need for anesthesia, no seizure induction, and a lack of significant cognitive side effects. The remission rates of daily left DLPFC are 15% (compared with 5% in a sham stimulation group).[174]

rTMS is well tolerated and most trials show high retention rates. The most reported side effects are discomfort caused by scalp or facial muscle twitching or headaches.[175] The most serious adverse effects reported with rTMS are seizures, but these have been unusual even when subjects were exposed to supratherapeutic parameters.[176,177]

With regards to the elderly population, rTMS is believed to be less effective than in younger patients. Compared with younger populations, the rates of response to rTMS are reported to be lower.[178] In a study conducted in 20 patients with an average age of

60 years, rTMS was not shown to be effective over sham stimulation. A drawback to this report is that the sample size was small and the dose of rTMS was nonthera-peutic.[179] The reason for the decreased efficacy may be related to diminished brain volumes (in particular frontal lobes), and white matter cerebrovascular lesions disrupt-ing the connections from DLPFC to mood-regulation subcortical centers.[180] On the other hand, an analysis by Lisanby and colleagues[181] did not find age to be a signif-icant predictor of response (clinical response between patients older or younger than 55 years were not significant). Positive predictors were found to be shorter dura-tion (<2 years) of the current depressive episode, degree of treatment resistance (≤1 treatment failure vs >1).

Deep Brain Stimulation

DBS is a well-established treatment of medication-refractory movement disorders, such as PD, essential tremor, and dystonia.[182–184] In the last decade, it has been increasingly explored for several psychiatric disorders, and a DBS system was recently granted FDA approval for the treatment of severe, treatment-resistant obsessive-compulsive disorder through a Humanitarian Device Exemption.[185] The mechanisms mediating DBS effects are more complex than a functional inhibition caused by high-frequency local stimulation, and there is evidence of both excitatory and inhibitory effects on brain regions adjacent to and remote from the site of stim-ulation.[186] Several brain regions are being investigated, with the highest number of patients implanted in the subcallosal cingulate area,[187–190] the nucleus accum-bens,[191,192] and the ventral capsule/ventral striatum.[193] Several randomized clinical trials are under way.[194] Preliminary reports are promising, and show good levels of clinical response across different targets.[195] The efficacy is sustained as long as stimulation is maintained and rates of response are between 40% and 75%, with follow-up periods of up to 6 years.[189] Other areas targeted for the treatment of depression with DBS are the lateral habenula,[196] the inferior thalamic peduncle,[197] and the medial forebrain bundle.[198] The procedure is the most invasive of the neuro-modulatory approaches discussed here, requiring neurosurgical implantation of bilat-eral electrodes in the selected area of interest. The complications associated with the neurosurgery involve hemorrhage, seizures, and infection, but these occur in low rates.[199] The patients receiving DBS for treatment-resistant depression were on average in their 40s at the time of implantation, so these results may not be immedi-ately extrapolated to the population with late-life depression. However, DBS for different indications, including PD, is being performed safely in patients older than 60 years, and trials are under way with implantation in the fornix and nucleus basalis of Meynert for the treatment of dementias.[200,201] DBS in the subcallosal cingulate white matter and in the nucleus accumbens has also been reported to be safe neuro-cognitively, even reporting improved cognitive effects that were not directly related to the improvement in mood.[202,203]

Transcranial Direct Current Stimulation

As discussed with rTMS, modulation of the DLPFC seems to generate positive results in the treatment of depression. In tDCS, delivery of weak electrical currents modulates the excitability of the cerebral cortex. Two sponge electrodes are placed in the skull, and current flows through the cortical area, and changes in brain-derived neurotrophic factor, cerebral blood flow, and metabolism have been reported.[204] A pivotal study by Fregni and colleagues,[205] as well as randomized double-blind trials by Boggio and col-leagues[206] and Loo and colleagues,[207] have reported preliminary efficacy compared with sham stimulation. This treatment approach is minimally invasive, inexpensive, and easy to use,[208] making it a promising alternative in patients with failures to other treatments. Tingling beneath the electrodes and, in some cases, minor skin burns have been reported. This treatment is still under investigational use, and the optimal parameters (polarity, current, ideal electrode placement, frequency and intensity of use) are yet to be defined.[209]

Magnetic Seizure Therapy

In MST, magnetic fields are used to induce therapeutic seizures. By using a more focal approach, seizures are induced in the prefrontal cortex, sparing mesial temporal structures, preventing cognitive side effects caused by ECT.[210] There have been several case reports and trials reporting the safety and efficacy of MST, with efficacy rates that are promising not only in improvement of depressive symptoms but also in neuropsychological assessments after treatment.[211]

Focal Electrically Administered Seizure Therapy

As in MST, with attempts to reduce the side effects from ECT and maintain its antidepressant efficacy, different approaches to the way the electrical current is delivered are being tried. Studies in nonhuman primates have shown the capacity to produce focal frontal seizure induction under conditions when a unidirectional current flows from a small anterior anode on the forehead to a large posterior cathode just anterior to the motor cortex. Therefore, FEAST combines unidirectional stimulation with a new electrode configuration in an attempt to enhance the efficiency and focality of seizure initiation.[212] Pilot studies are ongoing to investigate the safety and efficacy of FEAST.[213]

SUMMARY

Somatic nonpharmacological interventions, with ECT being the most evidence-based, safe, and validated by decades of clinical practice and research, are useful and essential options for treatment in the geriatric population with mood disorders. Newer approaches, most of them still experimental, are becoming more available, with significant differences in results, invasiveness, and side effect profiles. Focal neuromodulation strategies may in the next few years become accessible tools to use in the management of difficult-to-treat patients with severe mood disorders. Noninvasive strategies that do not require general anesthesia and are easily administered in the outpatient setting may be valuable adjuncts to the current treatment options. The most invasive methods, like DBS, seem to offer encouraging results for those patients who have failed the first-line and second-line treatments.

REFERENCES

1. Unutzer J, Park M. Older adults with severe, treatment-resistant depression. JAMA 2012;308(9):909–18.
2. Flint AJ. Treatment-resistant depression in late life. CNS Spectr 2002;7(10): 733–8.
3. Tew JD Jr, Mulsant BH, Haskett RF, et al. Acute efficacy of ECT in the treatment of major depression in the old-old. Am J Psychiatry 1999;156(12):1865–70.
4. Cattan RA, Barry PP, Mead G, et al. Electroconvulsive therapy in octogenarians. J Am Geriatr Soc 1990;38(7):753–8.
5. Sackeim HA, Prudic J, Fuller R, et al. The cognitive effects of electroconvulsive therapy in community settings. Neuropsychopharmacology 2007;32(1):244–54.

6. d'Elia G, Raotma H. Is unilateral ECT less effective than bilateral ECT? Br J Psychiatry 1975;126:83–9.

7. Letemendia FJ, Delva NJ, Rodenburg M, et al. Therapeutic advantage of bifrontal electrode placement in ECT. Psychol Med 1993;23(2):349–60.

8. Swartz CM. Asymmetric bilateral right frontotemporal left frontal stimulus electrode placement for electroconvulsive therapy. Neuropsychobiology 1994; 29(4):174–8.

9. Sackeim HA, Prudic J, Devanand DP, et al. Effects of stimulus intensity and electrode placement on the efficacy and cognitive effects of electroconvulsive therapy [see comments]. N Engl J Med 1993;328(12):839–46.

10. Sackeim HA, Prudic J, Devanand DP, et al. A prospective, randomized, double-blind comparison of bilateral and right unilateral electroconvulsive therapy at different stimulus intensities [see comments]. Arch Gen Psychiatry 2000;57(5): 425–34.

11. Damm J, Eser D, Schule C, et al. Influence of age on effectiveness and tolerability of electroconvulsive therapy. J ECT 2010;26(4):282–8.

12. van der Wurff FB, Stek ML, Hoogendijk WJ, et al. The efficacy and safety of ECT in depressed older adults: a literature review. Int J Geriatr Psychiatry 2003; 18(10):894–904.

13. Flint AJ, Gagnon N. Effective use of electroconvulsive therapy in late-life depression. Can J Psychiatry 2002;47(8):734–41.

14. Greenberg RM, Kellner CH. Electroconvulsive therapy: a selected review. Am J Geriatr Psychiatry 2005;13(4):268–81.

15. McCall WV, Cohen W, Reboussin B, et al. Pretreatment differences in specific symptoms and quality of life among depressed inpatients who do and do not receive electroconvulsive therapy: a hypothesis regarding why the elderly are more likely to receive ECT. J ECT 1999;15(3):193–201.

16. Ladwig KH, Klupsch D, Ruf E, et al. Sex- and age-related increase in prevalence rates of death wishes and suicidal ideation in the community: results from the KORA-F3 Augsburg Study with 3,154 men and women, 35 to 84 years of age. Psychiatry Res 2008;161(2):248–52.

17. Conwell Y, Brent D. Suicide and aging. I: patterns of psychiatric diagnosis. Int Psychogeriatr 1995;7(2):149–64.

18. Prudic J, Sackeim HA. Electroconvulsive therapy and suicide risk. J Clin Psychiatry 1999;60(Suppl 2):104–10 [discussion: 111–6].

19. Kellner CH, Fink M, Knapp R, et al. Relief of expressed suicidal intent by ECT: a consortium for research in ECT study. Am J Psychiatry 2005;162(5):977–82.

20. Patel M, Patel S, Hardy DW, et al. Should electroconvulsive therapy be an early consideration for suicidal patients? J ECT 2006;22(2):113–5.

21. Brodaty H, Luscombe G, Parker G, et al. Increased rate of psychosis and psychomotor change in depression with age. Psychol Med 1997;27(5): 1205–13.

22. Meyers BS, Klimstra SA, Gabriele M, et al. Continuation treatment of delusional depression in older adults. Am J Geriatr Psychiatry 2001;9(4):415–22.

23. Birkenhager TK, Pluijms EM, Lucius SA. ECT response in delusional versus nondelusional depressed inpatients. J Affect Disord 2003;74(2):191–5.

24. Petrides G, Fink M, Husain MM, et al. ECT remission rates in psychotic versus nonpsychotic depressed patients: a report from CORE. J ECT 2001;17(4): 244–53.

25. Aziz R, Lorberg B, Tampi RR. Treatments for late-life bipolar disorder. Am J Geriatr Pharmacother 2006;4(4):347–64.

26. Goldstein BI, Herrmann N, Shulman KI. Comorbidity in bipolar disorder among the elderly: results from an epidemiological community sample. Am J Psychiatry 2006;163(2):319–21.

27. Rosenzweig I, Earl H, Wai C, et al. Geriatric manic delirium with no previous history of mania. J Neuropsychiatry Clin Neurosci 2011;23(3):E39–41.

28. Ciapparelli A, Dell'Osso L, Tundo A, et al. Electroconvulsive therapy in medication-nonresponsive patients with mixed mania and bipolar depression. J Clin Psychiatry 2001;62(7):552–5.

29. Daly JJ, Prudic J, Devanand DP, et al. ECT in bipolar and unipolar depression: differences in speed of response. Bipolar Disord 2001;3(2):95–104.

30. Devanand DP, Polanco P, Cruz R, et al. The efficacy of ECT in mixed affective states. J ECT 2000;16(1):32–7.

31. Husain MM, Meyer DE, Muttakin MH, et al. Maintenance ECT for treatment of recurrent mania [letter]. Am J Psychiatry 1993;150(6):985.

32. Keck PE Jr, Mendlwicz J, Calabrese JR, et al. A review of randomized, controlled clinical trials in acute mania. J Affect Disord 2000;59(Suppl 1):S31–7.

33. Kho KH. Treatment of rapid cycling bipolar disorder in the acute and maintenance phase with ECT. J ECT 2002;18(3):159–61.

34. Macedo-Soares MB, Moreno RA, Rigonatti SP, et al. Efficacy of electroconvulsive therapy in treatment-resistant bipolar disorder: a case series. J ECT 2005;21(1):31–4.

35. Medda P, Perugi G, Zanello S, et al. Response to ECT in bipolar I, bipolar II and unipolar depression. J Affect Disord 2009;118(1–3):55–9.

36. Medda P, Perugi G, Zanello S, et al. Comparative response to electroconvulsive therapy in medication-resistant bipolar I patients with depression and mixed state. J ECT 2010;26(2):82–6.

37. Mukherjee S, Sackeim HA, Schnur DB. Electroconvulsive therapy of acute manic episodes: a review of 50 years' experience [see comments]. Am J Psychiatry 1994;151(2):169–76.

38. Poon SH, Sim K, Sum MY, et al. Evidence-based options for treatment-resistant adult bipolar disorder patients. Bipolar Disord 2012;14(6):573–84.

39. Robinson LA, Penzner JB, Arkow S, et al. Electroconvulsive therapy for the treatment of refractory mania. J Psychiatr Pract 2011;17(1):61–6.

40. Sachs GS, Printz DJ, Kahn DA, et al. The expert consensus guideline series: medication treatment of bipolar disorder 2000. Postgrad Med 2000;(Spec No):1–104.

41. Sienaert P, Peuskens J. Electroconvulsive therapy: an effective therapy of medication-resistant bipolar disorder. Bipolar Disord 2006;8(3):304–6.

42. Sienaert P, Vansteelandt K, Demyttenaere K, et al. Ultra-brief pulse ECT in bipolar and unipolar depressive disorder: differences in speed of response. Bipolar Disord 2009;11(4):418–24.

43. Tsao CI, Jain S, Gibson RH, et al. Maintenance ECT for recurrent medication-refractory mania. J ECT 2004;20(2):118–9.

44. Vaidya NA, Mahableshwarkar AR, Shahid R. Continuation and maintenance ECT in treatment-resistant bipolar disorder. J ECT 2003;19(1):10–6.

45. Vanelle JM, Loo H, Galinowski A, et al. Maintenance ECT in intractable manic-depressive disorders. Convuls Ther 1994;10(3):195–205.

46. Vieta E, Colom F. Therapeutic options in treatment-resistant depression. Ann Med 2011;43(7):512–30.

47. McDonald WM, Nemeroff CB. The diagnosis and treatment of mania in the elderly. Bull Menninger Clin 1996;60(2):174–96.

48. McDonald WM, Thompson TR. Treatment of mania in dementia with electroconvulsive therapy. Psychopharmacol Bull 2001;35(2):72–82.
49. Wilkins KM, Ostroff R, Tampi RR. Efficacy of electroconvulsive therapy in the treatment of nondepressed psychiatric illness in elderly patients: a review of the literature. J Geriatr Psychiatry Neurol 2008;21(1):3–11.
50. McDonald WM, Richard IH, DeLong MR. Prevalence, etiology, and treatment of depression in Parkinson's disease. Biol Psychiatry 2003;54(3):363–75.
51. Menza M, Dobkin RD, Marin H. Treatment of depression in Parkinson's disease. Curr Psychiatry Rep 2006;8(3):234–40.
52. McDonald WM, Holtzheimer PE 3rd, Byrd EH. The diagnosis and treatment of depression in Parkinson's disease. Curr Treat Options Neurol 2006;8(3): 245–55.
53. Baez MA, Avery J. Improvement in drug-induced parkinsonism with electroconvulsive therapy. Am J Geriatr Pharmacother 2011;9(3):190–3.
54. Fregni F, Simon DK, Wu A, et al. Non-invasive brain stimulation for Parkinson's disease: a systematic review and meta-analysis of the literature. J Neurol Neurosurg Psychiatr 2005;76(12):1614–23.
55. Popeo D, Kellner CH. ECT for Parkinson's disease. Med Hypotheses 2009;73(4): 468–9.
56. Aarsland D, Larsen JP, Waage O, et al. Maintenance electroconvulsive therapy for Parkinson's disease. Convuls Ther 1997;13(4):274–7.
57. McDonald W, Meeks T, McCall W, et al. Electroconvulsive therapy. In: Schatzberg AF, Nemeroff CB, editors. Textbook of psychopharmacology. 4th edition. Washington, DC: American Psychiatric Publishing; 2009. p. 861–902.
58. Mulsant BH, Rosen J, Thornton JE, et al. A prospective naturalistic study of electroconvulsive therapy in late-life depression. J Geriatr Psychiatry Neurol 1991; 4(1):3–13.
59. Hausner L, Damian M, Sartorius A, et al. Efficacy and cognitive side effects of electroconvulsive therapy (ECT) in depressed elderly inpatients with coexisting mild cognitive impairment or dementia. J Clin Psychiatry 2011;72(1):91–7.
60. Cohen-Mansfield J. Nonpharmacologic interventions for inappropriate behaviors in dementia: a review, summary, and critique. Am J Geriatr Psychiatry 2001;9(4):361–81.
61. Ballard C, Gray A, Ayre G. Psychotic symptoms, aggression and restlessness in dementia. Rev Neurol (Paris) 1999;155(Suppl 4):S44–52.
62. Ballard C, Walker M. Neuropsychiatric aspects of Alzheimer's disease. Curr Psychiatry Rep 1999;1(1):49–60.
63. Ballard CG, Shaw F, Lowery K, et al. The prevalence, assessment and associations of falls in dementia with Lewy bodies and Alzheimer's disease. Dement Geriatr Cogn Disord 1999;10(2):97–103.
64. Bartels SJ, Horn SD, Smout RJ, et al. Agitation and depression in frail nursing home elderly patients with dementia: treatment characteristics and service use. Am J Geriatr Psychiatry 2003;11(2):231–8.
65. Oudman E. Is electroconvulsive therapy (ECT) effective and safe for treatment of depression in dementia? A short review. J ECT 2012;28(1):34–8.
66. Ujkaj M, Davidoff DA, Seiner SJ, et al. Safety and efficacy of electroconvulsive therapy for the treatment of agitation and aggression in patients with dementia. Am J Geriatr Psychiatry 2012;20(1):61–72.
67. Weintraub D, Hurtig HI. Presentation and management of psychosis in Parkinson's disease and dementia with Lewy bodies. Am J Psychiatry 2007;164(10): 1491–8.

68. Takahashi S, Mizukami K, Yasuno F, et al. Depression associated with dementia with Lewy bodies (DLB) and the effect of somatotherapy. Psychogeriatrics 2009; 9(2):56–61.

69. Rasmussen KG Jr, Russell JC, Kung S, et al. Electroconvulsive therapy for patients with major depression and probable Lewy body dementia. J ECT 2003;19(2):103–9.

70. Hazzard WR, Ettinger WH Jr. Aging and atherosclerosis: changing considerations in cardiovascular disease prevention as the barrier to immortality is approached in old age. Am J Geriatr Cardiol 1995;4(4):16–36.

71. Sacco RL, Adams R, Albers G, et al. Guidelines for prevention of stroke in patients with ischemic stroke or transient ischemic attack: a statement for healthcare professionals from the American Heart Association/American Stroke Association Council on Stroke: co-sponsored by the Council on Cardiovascular Radiology and Intervention: the American Academy of Neurology affirms the value of this guideline. Stroke 2006;37(2):577–617.

72. Lokk J, Delbari A. Management of depression in elderly stroke patients. Neuropsychiatr Dis Treat 2010;6:539–49.

73. Hackett ML, Anderson CS, House A, et al. Interventions for treating depression after stroke. Cochrane Database Syst Rev 2008;(4):CD003437.

74. DeQuardo JR, Tandon R. ECT in post-stroke major depression. Convuls Ther 1988;4(3):221–4.

75. Murray GB, Shea V, Conn DK. Electroconvulsive therapy for poststroke depression. J Clin Psychiatry 1986;47(5):258–60.

76. Currier MB, Murray GB, Welch CC. Electroconvulsive therapy for post-stroke depressed geriatric patients. J Neuropsychiatry Clin Neurosci 1992;4(2):140–4.

77. Weintraub D, Lippmann SB. Electroconvulsive therapy in the acute poststroke period. J ECT 2000;16(4):415–8.

78. Harmandayan M, Romanowicz M, Sola C. Successful use of ECT in post-stroke depression. Gen Hosp Psychiatry 2012;34(1):102.e5–6.

79. Miller AR, Isenberg KE. Reversible ischemic neurologic deficit after ECT. J ECT 1998;14(1):42–8.

80. Bruce BB, Henry ME, Greer DM. Ischemic stroke after electroconvulsive therapy. J ECT 2006;22(2):150–2.

81. Weisberg LA, Elliott D, Mielke D. Intracerebral hemorrhage following electroconvulsive therapy. Neurology 1991;41(11):1849.

82. Pritchett J, Kellner C, Coffey C. Electroconvulsive therapy in geriatric neuropsychiatry. In: Coffey CE, Cummings JL, editors. Textbook of geriatric neuropsychiatry. Washington, DC: American Psychiatric Press; 1994. p. 650–1.

83. Gazdag G, Takacs R, Ungvari GS, et al. The practice of consenting to electroconvulsive therapy in the European Union. J ECT 2012;28(1):4–6.

84. Amazon J, McNeely E, Lehr S, et al. The decision making process of older adults who elect to receive ECT. J Psychosoc Nurs Ment Health Serv 2008; 46(5):45–52.

85. Brodaty H, Hickie I, Mason C, et al. A prospective follow-up study of ECT outcome in older depressed patients. J Affect Disord 2000;60(2):101–11.

86. Lapid MI, Rummans TA, Pankratz VS, et al. Decisional capacity of depressed elderly to consent to electroconvulsive therapy. J Geriatr Psychiatry Neurol 2004;17(1):42–6.

87. Chakrabarti S, Grover S, Rajagopal R. Perceptions and awareness of electroconvulsive therapy among patients and their families: a review of the research from developing countries. J ECT 2010;26(4):317–22.

88. Lapid MI, Rummans TA, Poole KL, et al. Decisional capacity of severely depressed patients requiring electroconvulsive therapy. J ECT 2003;19(2): 67–72.

89. Tang WK, Ungvari GS, Chan GW. Patients' and their relatives' knowledge of, experience with, attitude toward, and satisfaction with electroconvulsive therapy in Hong Kong, China. J ECT 2002;18(4):207–12.

90. Task Force Report of the American Psychiatric Association. The practice of electroconvulsive therapy: recommendations for treatment, training and privileging. In: Weiner RD, editor. Task force report on ECT. 2nd edition. Washington, DC: American Psychiatric Association; 2001.

91. Akcaboy ZN, Akcaboy EY, Yigitbasl B, et al. Effects of remifentanil and alfentanil on seizure duration, stimulus amplitudes and recovery parameters during ECT. Acta Anaesthesiol Scand 2005;49(8):1068–71.

92. Avramov MN, Husain MM, White PF. The comparative effects of methohexital, propofol, and etomidate for electroconvulsive therapy. Anesth Analg 1995; 81(3):596–602.

93. Badrinath S, Avramov MN, Shadrick M, et al. The use of a ketamine-propofol combination during monitored anesthesia care. Anesth Analg 2000;90(4): 858–62.

94. Krystal AD, Watts BV, Weiner RD, et al. The use of flumazenil in the anxious and benzodiazepine-dependent ECT patient. J ECT 1998;14(1):5–14.

95. Gilabert E, Rojo E, Vallejo J. Augmentation of electroconvulsive therapy seizures with sleep deprivation. J ECT 2004;20(4):242–7.

96. Sawayama E, Takahashi M, Inoue A, et al. Moderate hyperventilation prolongs electroencephalogram seizure duration of the first electroconvulsive therapy. J ECT 2008;24(3):195–8.

97. Cristancho MA, Alici Y, Augoustides JG, et al. Uncommon but serious complications associated with electroconvulsive therapy: recognition and management for the clinician. Curr Psychiatry Rep 2008;10(6):474–80.

98. Zielinski RJ, Roose SP, Devanand DP, et al. Cardiovascular complications of ECT in depressed patients with cardiac disease. Am J Psychiatry 1993; 150(6):904–9.

99. Figiel GS, McDonald WM, McCall WV, et al. Electroconvulsive therapy. In: Schatzberg AF, Nemeroff CB, editors. Textbook of psychopharmacology. Washington, DC: American Psychiatric Press; 1995. p. 523–43.

100. Avramov MN, Stool LA, White PF, et al. Effects of nicardipine and labetalol on the acute hemodynamic response to electroconvulsive therapy. J Clin Anesth 1998; 10(5):394–400.

101. Zhang Y, White PF, Thornton L, et al. The use of nicardipine for electroconvulsive therapy: a dose-ranging study. Anesth Analg 2005;100(2):378–81.

102. Kokras N, Politis AM, Zervas IM, et al. Cardiac rhythm management devices and electroconvulsive therapy: a critical review apropos of a depressed patient with a pacemaker. J ECT 2011;27(3):214–20.

103. Dolenc TJ, Barnes RD, Hayes DL, et al. Electroconvulsive therapy in patients with cardiac pacemakers and implantable cardioverter defibrillators. Pacing Clin Electrophysiol 2004;27(9):1257–63.

104. Giltay EJ, Kho KH, Keijzer LT, et al. Electroconvulsive therapy (ECT) in a patient with a dual-chamber sensing, VDDR pacemaker. J ECT 2005;21(1):35–8.

105. Petrides G, Fink M. Atrial fibrillation, anticoagulation, and electroconvulsive therapy. Convuls Ther 1996;12(2):91–8.

106. Gardner M, Kellner MD, Hood D, et al. The safe administration of ECT in a patient with a cardiac aneurysm and multiple cardiac risk factors. Convuls Ther 1997;13(3):200–3.

107. Porquez JM, Thompson TR, McDonald WM. Administration of ECT in a patient with an inoperable abdominal aortic aneurysm: serial imaging of the aorta during maintenance. J ECT 2003;19(2):118–20.

108. Pomeranze J, Karliner W, Triebel WA, et al. Electroshock therapy in presence of serious organic disease. Depression and aortic aneurysm. Geriatrics 1968; 23(10):122–4.

109. Najjar F, Guttmacher LB. ECT in the presence of intracranial aneurysm. J ECT 1998;14(4):266–71.

110. Boey WK, Lai FO. Comparison of propofol and thiopentone as anaesthetic agents for electroconvulsive therapy. Anaesthesia 1990;45(8):623–8.

111. Rosa MA, Rosa MO, Belegarde IM, et al. Recovery after ECT: comparison of propofol, etomidate and thiopental. Rev Bras Psiquiatr 2008;30(2):149–51.

112. Hermida A, McClam T, Syre S, et al. Prevention of post-ictal agitation after electroconvulsive therapy. Poster session presented at the ISEN annual meeting. Philadelphia, May 7, 2012.

113. Sackeim HA, Luber B, Moeller JR, et al. Electrophysiological correlates of the adverse cognitive effects of electroconvulsive therapy. J ECT 2000;16(2): 110–20.

114. Deng ZD, Lisanby SH, Peterchev AV. Electric field strength and focality in electroconvulsive therapy and magnetic seizure therapy: a finite element simulation study. J Neural Eng 2011;8(1):016007.

115. Fujita A, Nakaaki S, Segawa K, et al. Memory, attention, and executive functions before and after sine and pulse wave electroconvulsive therapies for treatment-resistant major depression. J ECT 2006;22(2):107–12.

116. Hyrman V. Pulse width and frequency in ECT. J ECT 1999;15(4):285–90.

117. Loo CK, Sainsbury K, Sheehan P, et al. A comparison of RUL ultrabrief pulse (0.3 ms) ECT and standard RUL ECT. Int J Neuropsychopharmacol 2008; 11(7):883–90.

118. Sackeim HA, Prudic J, Nobler MS, et al. Effects of pulse width and electrode placement on the efficacy and cognitive effects of electroconvulsive therapy. Brain Stimul 2008;1(2):71–83.

119. Sienaert P, Vansteelandt K, Demyttenaere K, et al. Randomized comparison of ultra-brief bifrontal and unilateral electroconvulsive therapy for major depression: cognitive side-effects. J Affect Disord 2010;122(1–2):60–7.

120. Petrides G, Braga RJ, Fink M, et al. Seizure threshold in a large sample: implications for stimulus dosing strategies in bilateral electroconvulsive therapy: a report from CORE. J ECT 2009;25(4):232–7.

121. Coffey CE, Lucke J, Weiner RD, et al. Seizure threshold in electroconvulsive therapy: I. Initial seizure threshold. Biol Psychiatry 1995;37(10):713–20.

122. McCall WV, Reboussin DM, Weiner RD, et al. Titrated moderately suprathreshold vs fixed high-dose right unilateral electroconvulsive therapy: acute antidepressant and cognitive effects [see comments]. Arch Gen Psychiatry 2000;57(5): 438–44.

123. Quante A, Luborzewski A, Brakemeier EL, et al. Effects of 3 different stimulus intensities of ultrabrief stimuli in right unilateral electroconvulsive therapy in major depression: a randomized, double-blind pilot study. J Psychiatr Res 2011;45(2):174–8.

124. Bennett DM, Perrin JS, Currie J, et al. A comparison of ECT dosing methods using a clinical sample. J Affect Disord 2012;141(2–3):222–6.
125. Petrides G, Braga RJ, Fink M, et al. Stimulus dosing in electroconvulsive therapy. J ECT 2011;27(3):268.
126. Prudic J, Sackeim HA, Devanand DP, et al. Acute cognitive effects of subconvulsive electrical stimulation. Convuls Ther 1994;10(1):4–24.
127. Hermida A, Stair S, Zhao L, et al. Initial stimulus dosing in ECT: a comparison between seizure titration with other predictive dosing strategies. Poster session at the 2012 National Network of Depression Centers Conference. Rochester, November 8, 2012.
128. Figiel GS, McDonald WM, McCall WV, et al. Electroconvulsive therapy. In: Schatzberg AF, Nemeroff CB, editors. Textbook of psychopharmacology. 2nd edition. Washington, DC: American Psychiatric Press; 1998. p. 523–4.
129. Folstein MF, Folstein SE, McHugh PR. "Mini-mental state". A practical method for grading the cognitive state of patients for the clinician. J Psychiatr Res 1975; 12(3):189–98.
130. Steif BL, Sackeim HA, Portnoy S, et al. Effects of depression and ECT on anterograde memory. Biol Psychiatry 1986;21(10):921–30.
131. Prudic J, Peyser S, Sackeim HA. Subjective memory complaints: a review of patient self-assessment of memory after electroconvulsive therapy [see comments]. J ECT 2000;16(2):121–32.
132. Lisanby SH, Maddox JH, Prudic J, et al. The effects of electroconvulsive therapy on memory of autobiographical and public events. Arch Gen Psychiatry 2000; 57(6):581–90.
133. Stoppe A, Louza M, Rosa M, et al. Fixed high-dose electroconvulsive therapy in the elderly with depression: a double-blind, randomized comparison of efficacy and tolerability between unilateral and bilateral electrode placement. J ECT 2006;22(2):92–9.
134. Kellner CH, Knapp R, Husain MM, et al. Bifrontal, bitemporal and right unilateral electrode placement in ECT: randomised trial. Br J Psychiatry 2010;196(3): 226–34.
135. Sobin C, Sackeim HA, Prudic J, et al. Predictors of retrograde amnesia following ECT. Am J Psychiatry 1995;152(7):995–1001.
136. Lerer B, Shapira B, Calev A, et al. Antidepressant and cognitive effects of twice- versus three-times-weekly ECT. Am J Psychiatry 1995;152(4):564–70.
137. Krueger RB, Sackeim HA, Gamzu ER. Pharmacological treatment of the cognitive side effects of ECT: a review. Psychopharmacol Bull 1992;28(4):409–24.
138. Prudic J, Fitzsimons L, Nobler MS, et al. Naloxone in the prevention of the adverse cognitive effects of ECT: a within-subject, placebo controlled study. Neuropsychopharmacology 1999;21(2):285–93.
139. Prakash J, Kotwal A, Prabhu H. Therapeutic and prophylactic utility of the memory-enhancing drug donepezil hydrochloride on cognition of patients undergoing electroconvulsive therapy: a randomized controlled trial. J ECT 2006;22(3):163–8.
140. Matthews JD, Blais M, Park L, et al. The impact of galantamine on cognition and mood during electroconvulsive therapy: a pilot study. J Psychiatr Res 2008; 42(7):526–31.
141. Kellner CH, Knapp RG, Petrides G, et al. Continuation electroconvulsive therapy vs pharmacotherapy for relapse prevention in major depression: a multisite study from the Consortium for Research in Electroconvulsive Therapy (CORE). Arch Gen Psychiatry 2006;63(12):1337–44.

142. Rapinesi C, Kotzalidis GD, Serata D, et al. Prevention of relapse with maintenance electroconvulsive therapy in elderly patients with major depressive episode. J ECT 2013;29(1):61–4.

143. Rabheru K. Maintenance electroconvulsive therapy (M-ECT) after acute response: examining the evidence for who, what, when, and how? J ECT 2012;28(1):39–47.

144. van Schaik AM, Comijs HC, Sonnenberg CM, et al. Efficacy and safety of continuation and maintenance electroconvulsive therapy in depressed elderly patients: a systematic review. Am J Geriatr Psychiatry 2012;20(1):5–17.

145. Trevino K, McClintock SM, Husain MM. A review of continuation electroconvulsive therapy: application, safety, and efficacy. J ECT 2010;26(3):186–95.

146. McDonald WM, Phillips VL, Figiel GS, et al. Cost-effective maintenance treatment of resistant geriatric depression. Psychiatr Ann 1998;28(1):47–52.

147. McDonald WM. Is ECT cost-effective? A critique of the National Institute of Health and Clinical Excellence's report on the economic analysis of ECT. J ECT 2006;22(1):25–9.

148. Nordenskjold A, von Knorring L, Ljung T, et al. Continuation electroconvulsive therapy with pharmacotherapy versus pharmacotherapy alone for prevention of relapse of depression: a randomized controlled trial. J ECT 2013;29(2):86–92.

149. Nordenskjold A, von Knorring L, Engstrom I. Rehospitalization rate after continued electroconvulsive therapy–a retrospective chart review of patients with severe depression. Nord J Psychiatry 2011;65(1):26–31.

150. Huuhka K, Viikki M, Tammentie T, et al. One-year follow-up after discontinuing maintenance electroconvulsive therapy. J ECT 2012;28(4):225–8.

151. Sackeim HA, Haskett RF, Mulsant BH, et al. Continuation pharmacotherapy in the prevention of relapse following electroconvulsive therapy: a randomized controlled trial [see comments]. JAMA 2001;285(10):1299–307.

152. Tew JD Jr, Mulsant BH, Haskett RF, et al. Relapse during continuation pharmacotherapy after acute response to ECT: a comparison of usual care versus protocolized treatment. Ann Clin Psychiatry 2007;19(1):1–4.

153. Prudic J, Haskett RF, McCall WV, et al. Pharmacological strategies in the prevention of relapse after electroconvulsive therapy. J ECT 2013;29(1):3–12.

154. Sartorius A, Wolf J, Henn FA. Lithium and ECT–concurrent use still demands attention: three case reports. World J Biol Psychiatry 2005;6(2):121–4.

155. Small JG, Kellams JJ, Milstein V, et al. Complications with electroconvulsive treatment combined with lithium. Biol Psychiatry 1980;15(1):103–12.

156. Small JG, Milstein V. Lithium interactions: lithium and electroconvulsive therapy. J Clin Psychopharmacol 1990;10(5):346–50.

157. Weiner RD, Whanger AD, Erwin CW, et al. Prolonged confusional state and EEG seizure activity following concurrent ECT and lithium use. Am J Psychiatry 1980; 137(11):1452–3.

158. Mukherjee S. Combined ECT and lithium therapy. Convuls Ther 1993;9(4): 274–84.

159. Stewart JT. Lithium and maintenance ECT. J ECT 2000;16(3):300–1.

160. Mayberg HS. Limbic-cortical dysregulation: a proposed model of depression. J Neuropsychiatry Clin Neurosci 1997;9(3):471–81.

161. Mayberg HS. Modulating dysfunctional limbic-cortical circuits in depression: towards development of brain-based algorithms for diagnosis and optimised treatment. Br Med Bull 2003;65:193–207.

162. Elger G, Hoppe C, Falkai P, et al. Vagus nerve stimulation is associated with mood improvements in epilepsy patients. Epilepsy Res 2000;42(2–3):203–10.

163. Harden CL, Pulver MC, Ravdin LD, et al. A pilot study of mood in epilepsy patients treated with vagus nerve stimulation. Epilepsy Behav 2000;1(2): 93–9.

164. Dietrich DE, Emrich HM. The use of anticonvulsants to augment antidepressant medication. J Clin Psychiatry 1998;59(Suppl 5):51–8 [discussion: 59].

165. Krahl SE, Senanayake SS, Pekary AE, et al. Vagus nerve stimulation (VNS) is effective in a rat model of antidepressant action. J Psychiatr Res 2004;38(3): 237–40.

166. George MS, Sackeim HA, Marangell LB, et al. Vagus nerve stimulation. A potential therapy for resistant depression? Psychiatr Clin North Am 2000;23(4): 757–83.

167. Rush AJ, Marangell LB, Sackeim HA, et al. Vagus nerve stimulation for treatment-resistant depression: a randomized, controlled acute phase trial. Biol Psychiatry 2005;58(5):347–54.

168. Rush AJ, Sackeim HA, Marangell LB, et al. Effects of 12 months of vagus nerve stimulation in treatment-resistant depression: a naturalistic study. Biol Psychiatry 2005;58(5):355–63.

169. Sackeim HA, Brannan SK, Rush AJ, et al. Durability of antidepressant response to vagus nerve stimulation (VNS). Int J Neuropsychopharmacol 2007;10(6): 817–26.

170. Sirven JI, Sperling M, Naritoku D, et al. Vagus nerve stimulation therapy for epilepsy in older adults. Neurology 2000;54(5):1179–82.

171. Merrill CA, Jonsson MA, Minthon L, et al. Vagus nerve stimulation in patients with Alzheimer's disease: additional follow-up results of a pilot study through 1 year. J Clin Psychiatry 2006;67(8):1171–8.

172. O'Reardon JP, Solvason HB, Janicak PG, et al. Efficacy and safety of transcranial magnetic stimulation in the acute treatment of major depression: a multisite randomized controlled trial. Biol Psychiatry 2007;62(11):1208–16.

173. Schutter DJ. Quantitative review of the efficacy of slow-frequency magnetic brain stimulation in major depressive disorder. Psychol Med 2010;40(11): 1789–95.

174. George MS, Lisanby SH, Avery D, et al. Daily left prefrontal transcranial magnetic stimulation therapy for major depressive disorder: a sham-controlled randomized trial. Arch Gen Psychiatry 2010;67(5):507–16.

175. Burt T, Lisanby SH, Sackeim HA. Neuropsychiatric applications of transcranial magnetic stimulation: a meta analysis. Int J Neuropsychopharmacol 2002; 5(1):73–103.

176. Anderson B, Mishory A, Nahas Z, et al. Tolerability and safety of high daily doses of repetitive transcranial magnetic stimulation in healthy young men. J ECT 2006;22(1):49–53.

177. Wassermann EM. Risk and safety of repetitive transcranial magnetic stimulation: report and suggested guidelines from the International Workshop on the Safety of Repetitive Transcranial Magnetic Stimulation, June 5–7, 1996. Electroencephalogr Clin Neurophysiol 1998;108(1):1–16.

178. Figiel GS, Epstein C, McDonald WM, et al. The use of rapid-rate transcranial magnetic stimulation (rTMS) in refractory depressed patients. J Neuropsychiatry Clin Neurosci 1998;10(1):20–5.

179. Manes F, Jorge R, Morcuende M, et al. A controlled study of repetitive transcranial magnetic stimulation as a treatment of depression in the elderly. Int Psychogeriatr 2001;13(2):225–31.

180. Jalenques I, Legrand G, Vaille-Perret E, et al. Therapeutic efficacy and safety of repetitive transcranial magnetic stimulation in depressions of the elderly: a review. Encephale 2010;36(Suppl 2):D105–18 [in French].
181. Lisanby SH, Husain MM, Rosenquist PB, et al. Daily left prefrontal repetitive transcranial magnetic stimulation in the acute treatment of major depression: clinical predictors of outcome in a multisite, randomized controlled clinical trial. Neuropsychopharmacology 2009;34(2):522–34.
182. Toda H, Hamani C, Lozano A. Deep brain stimulation in the treatment of dyskinesia and dystonia. Neurosurg Focus 2004;17(1):E2.
183. Benabid AL, Pollak P, Louveau A, et al. Combined (thalamotomy and stimulation) stereotactic surgery of the VIM thalamic nucleus for bilateral Parkinson disease. Appl Neurophysiol 1987;50(1–6):344–6.
184. Lyons KE, Pahwa R. Deep brain stimulation and essential tremor. J Clin Neurophysiol 2004;21(1):2–5.
185. Food and Drug Administration, editor. Reclaim DBS therapy for OCD-H050003. Maryland: FDA; 2009.
186. Vitek JL. Mechanisms of deep brain stimulation: excitation or inhibition. Mov Disord 2002;17(Suppl 3):S69–72.
187. Holtzheimer PE, Kelley ME, Gross RE, et al. Subcallosal cingulate deep brain stimulation for treatment-resistant unipolar and bipolar depression. Arch Gen Psychiatry 2012;69(2):150–8.
188. Lozano AM, Mayberg HS, Giacobbe P, et al. Subcallosal cingulate gyrus deep brain stimulation for treatment-resistant depression. Biol Psychiatry 2008;64(6): 461–7.
189. Kennedy SH, Giacobbe P, Rizvi SJ, et al. Deep brain stimulation for treatment-resistant depression: follow-up after 3 to 6 years. Am J Psychiatry 2011;168(5): 502–10.
190. Puigdemont D, Perez-Egea R, Portella MJ, et al. Deep brain stimulation of the subcallosal cingulate gyrus: further evidence in treatment-resistant major depression. Int J Neuropsychopharmacol 2011;1–13.
191. Bewernick BH, Hurlemann R, Matusch A, et al. Nucleus accumbens deep brain stimulation decreases ratings of depression and anxiety in treatment-resistant depression. Biol Psychiatry 2010;67(2):110–6.
192. Bewernick BH, Kayser S, Sturm V, et al. Long-term effects of nucleus accumbens deep brain stimulation in treatment-resistant depression: evidence for sustained efficacy. Neuropsychopharmacology 2012;37(9): 1975–85.
193. Malone DA Jr, Dougherty DD, Rezai AR, et al. Deep brain stimulation of the ventral capsule/ventral striatum for treatment-resistant depression. Biol Psychiatry 2009;65(4):267–75.
194. Lozano AM, Giacobbe P, Hamani C, et al. A multicenter pilot study of subcallosal cingulate area deep brain stimulation for treatment-resistant depression. J Neurosurg 2012;116(2):315–22.
195. Riva-Posse P, Holtzheimer PE, Garlow SJ, et al. Practical considerations in the development and refinement of subcallosal cingulate white matter deep brain stimulation for treatment resistant depression. World Neurosurg 2012. [Epub ahead of print]. http://dx.doi.org/10.1016/j.wneu.2012.11.074.
196. Sartorius A, Kiening KL, Kirsch P, et al. Remission of major depression under deep brain stimulation of the lateral habenula in a therapy-refractory patient. Biol Psychiatry 2010;67(2):e9–11.

197. Jimenez F, Velasco F, Salin-Pascual R, et al. A patient with a resistant major depression disorder treated with deep brain stimulation in the inferior thalamic peduncle. Neurosurgery 2005;57(3):585–93 [discussion: 585–93].

198. Coenen VA, Schlaepfer TE, Maedler B, et al. Cross-species affective functions of the medial forebrain bundle-implications for the treatment of affective pain and depression in humans. Neurosci Biobehav Rev 2011;35(9):1971–81.

199. Blomstedt P, Sjoberg RL, Hansson M, et al. Deep brain stimulation in the treatment of depression. Acta Psychiatr Scand 2011;123(1):4–11.

200. Laxton AW, Lozano AM. Deep brain stimulation for the treatment of Alzheimer disease and dementias. World Neurosurg 2012. [Epub ahead of print]. http://dx.doi.org/10.1016/j.wneu.2012.06.028.

201. Laxton AW, Tang-Wai DF, McAndrews MP, et al. A phase I trial of deep brain stimulation of memory circuits in Alzheimer's disease. Ann Neurol 2010;68(4):521–34.

202. Moreines JL, McClintock SM, Holtzheimer PE. Neuropsychologic effects of neuromodulation techniques for treatment-resistant depression: a review. Brain Stimul 2011;4(1):17–27.

203. Grubert C, Hurlemann R, Bewernick BH, et al. Neuropsychological safety of nucleus accumbens deep brain stimulation for major depression: effects of 12-month stimulation. World J Biol Psychiatry 2011;12(7):516–27.

204. Fritsch B, Reis J, Martinowich K, et al. Direct current stimulation promotes BDNF-dependent synaptic plasticity: potential implications for motor learning. Neuron 2010;66(2):198–204.

205. Fregni F, Boggio PS, Nitsche MA, et al. Treatment of major depression with transcranial direct current stimulation. Bipolar Disord 2006;8(2):203–4.

206. Boggio PS, Rigonatti SP, Ribeiro RB, et al. A randomized, double-blind clinical trial on the efficacy of cortical direct current stimulation for the treatment of major depression. Int J Neuropsychopharmacol 2008;11(2):249–54.

207. Loo CK, Sachdev P, Martin D, et al. A double-blind, sham-controlled trial of transcranial direct current stimulation for the treatment of depression. Int J Neuropsychopharmacol 2010;13(1):61–9.

208. Dell'Osso B, Priori A, Altamura AC. Efficacy and safety of transcranial direct current stimulation in major depression. Biol Psychiatry 2011;69(8):e23–4.

209. Minhas P, Bansal V, Patel J, et al. Electrodes for high-definition transcutaneous DC stimulation for applications in drug delivery and electrotherapy, including tDCS. J Neurosci Methods 2010;190(2):188–97.

210. Lisanby SH, Luber B, Schlaepfer TE, et al. Safety and feasibility of magnetic seizure therapy (MST) in major depression: randomized within-subject comparison with electroconvulsive therapy. Neuropsychopharmacology 2003;28(10):1852–65.

211. Kayser S, Bewernick B, Axmacher N, et al. Magnetic seizure therapy of treatment-resistant depression in a patient with bipolar disorder. J ECT 2009;25(2):137–40.

212. Spellman T, Peterchev AV, Lisanby SH. Focal electrically administered seizure therapy: a novel form of ECT illustrates the roles of current directionality, polarity, and electrode configuration in seizure induction. Neuropsychopharmacology 2009;34(8):2002–10.

213. Nahas Z. Focal Electroconvulsive Therapy for Depression (FEAST). 2012. Available at: http://clinicaltrials.gov/. Accessed December 15, 2012.

The Economic, Public Health, and Caregiver Burden of Late-life Depression

Kara Zivin, PhD[a,b,c],*, Tracy Wharton, PhD[b], Ola Rostant, PhD[b]

KEYWORDS

- Late-life depression • Costs • Caregiver burden • Retirement • Public health

KEY POINTS

- Depression is a significant public health problem for older adults.
- There are multiple burdens of late-life depression (LLD) on patients, caregivers, and society.
- Basic, clinical, epidemiologic, and health services research should focus more resources and attention on this devastating and costly yet treatable illness.

OVERVIEW

Depression is a significant public health problem for older adults, yet many mistakenly think that depression is a normal part of aging.[1] Reports indicate that 15% to 27% of older adults in the community[2] and up to 37% in primary care settings[1] experience depressive symptoms. Subclinical (eg, nonmajor) depression is more prevalent in elderly populations than major depressive disorder (MDD). Depression in older adults, often identified as LLD, seems to differ from depression earlier in life, with increased heterogeneity across the adult population. Factors, such as age of onset, number of lifetime episodes, somatic symptoms, and comorbidities, all may contribute to or result from psychopathology.[3] Rates of depression have risen over the past decade,[4]

Funding Support and Disclosures: This study was funded by the Department of Veterans Affairs (VA IIR 10-176-3; Dr Zivin) and the Department of Veterans Affairs Health Services Research and Development Services (CD2 07-206-1; Dr Zivin). Drs Wharton and Rostant were funded by a National Institute of Mental Health T32 Geriatric Mental Health Services fellowship. The authors have no conflicts of interest to disclose.
[a] Serious Mental Illness Treatment Resource and Evaluation Center, Center for Clinical Management Research, Department of Veterans Affairs, Plymouth Road, Ann Arbor, MI 48109, USA; [b] Department of Psychiatry, University of Michigan Medical School, Plymouth Road, Ann Arbor, MI 48109, USA; [c] Institute for Social Research, University of Michigan Medical School, Thompson Street, Ann Arbor, MI 48104, USA
* Corresponding author. University of Michigan North Campus Research Complex, 2800 Plymouth Road, Building 16, Room 228W, Ann Arbor, MI 48109-2800.
E-mail address: kzivin@umich.edu

Psychiatr Clin N Am 36 (2013) 631–649
http://dx.doi.org/10.1016/j.psc.2013.08.008
0193-953X/13/$ – see front matter Published by Elsevier Inc.

suggesting that future cohorts of older adults will see higher numbers of individuals with depressive disorders.[5] As the US population ages, additional efforts will be needed to minimize the burden of depression for older adults and their loved ones.[6] Although LLD is associated with a substantial individual and societal burden, it receives much less attention than many medical disorders experienced by older adults.[7] Depression has a major impact on the use of medical services, daily functioning, and overall quality of life in later life.[8] Given the effects of depression on daily functioning, understanding ways to preserve mental health into late life assumes great importance.[6]

This article reviews the economic, public health, and caregiver burden of LLD, focusing primarily on the impact of depression rather than on risk factors for developing depression. The authors, however, present an example of the bidirectional relationship between depression and retirement among older adults to illustrate the complexity that can be associated with trying to disentangle the impact of depression on economic and public health outcomes.

The burden of depression is assessed from several perspectives, including economic, public health, and caregiver. Direct costs of depression include costs of depression treatment as well as treatment of other comorbid psychiatric and medical conditions. Indirect costs of depression include its impact on job functioning, disability, and retirement. This article considers these direct and indirect costs as the economic burden of LLD. Depression can lead to the onset and exacerbation of medical illness and even lead to death; this is considered the public health burden of LLD. Finally, LLD has an impact on others close to the patient, such as family members and caregivers. This burden is considered the caregiving burden for depression (which elsewhere has been considered another indirect cost).[9]

PREVALENCE AND PATTERNS OF LLD

Approximately 5 million adults age 65 and older experience LLD,[10] and LLD diagnoses have increased over time.[11] Yet in clinical practice LLD is often under-recognized and undertreated. Primary care physicians seem less successful in identifying depression in older people than in younger adults, although there have been few head-to-head studies stratified by age.[12]

Depression does not develop uniformly over the lifespan. Many analyses compare cross-sectional assessments of depression across age groups rather than longitudinal assessments of depression status,[13] although research on LLD trajectories has been increasing.[13–21] Recent research has identified several LLD trends of interest. Wu and colleagues[13] found that an age-related increase of depression symptoms occurs entirely through the relationship with medical illness, such as dementia, chronic conditions, and functional limitations. Once these risk factors are controlled, the relationship between age and depressive symptoms becomes nonsignificant. Other studies have found several distinct patterns of LLD depressive symptoms over time, including high or low levels of persistent symptoms[22] or remitting, intermittent, and chronic courses,[14] with variations by age and birth cohort.[16] These studies demonstrate the variability and diversity in patient experiences of LLD. Continued research into understanding subtypes, trajectories, and patterns of LLD may reveal important targets for future prevention, treatment, and intervention.

ECONOMIC BURDEN OF LLD
Direct Costs

Depression is among the top 10 most costly diseases in the United States,[23] comparable to physical illnesses.[24] Although some patients may first experience depression in later life, depression typically has an earlier age of onset than other major illnesses, leading to health care costs that accumulate over a long period of time. Depression is the leading cause of psychiatric hospitalizations in older adults.[25] It is associated with increased medical burden, health service utilization, longer hospital stays, disability, and more functional impairment than most medical disorders; however, most research is on younger age groups.[26] Given that depressed people, in particular older adults, consume health services and medical resources at a rate beyond that which can be explained by their depression alone (eg, they use more care for other medical disorders), depressed individuals place a substantial burden on societal resources.[27–31] Use of medical services by depressed patients exceeds that of similar nondepressed patients by 50% to 100%.[32–34]

Several studies have found variation in health care use based on depression severity. Goldney and colleagues[35] found the least use among the nondepressed, moderate use among those with subclinical depression, and the most use among those with MDD. Another study found that total health care costs rose with increasing depression severity.[36] An equal or greater burden can be attributed to depressive symptoms; although they are less costly than MDD, their higher prevalence[6] results in greater total societal costs.[28]

Fewer studies have assessed utilization patterns of elderly patients, yet LLD is associated with high utilization in many categories of medical care, not just mental health care, including inappropriate service use.[26] Excess costs of depression in community-dwelling elderly are significant even when productivity losses are not considered.[37] Depression in geriatric populations can present similarly or exacerbate somatic symptoms associated with comorbid medical conditions,[31] which can delay depression treatment.[38] Depressed elderly individuals with chronic medical conditions visit a doctor's office, visit an emergency department,[5] and are hospitalized[39] more frequently than their nondepressed counterparts.[40] Up to 25% of costs of care for medical illnesses may be attributed to depression, and this is clearly associated with longer hospital stays and higher costs.[41]

Health care costs, like utilization patterns, are significantly greater among older depressed patients.[29,42,43] Depressed Medicare enrollees have higher costs in every category of health care except for mental health specialty care.[42] Even after initiation of treatment, their health care costs are double that of their nondepressed counterparts.[34] Attempts to cut costs by limiting outpatient mental health care may not reduce overall costs, because mental health care comprises only a small proportion of overall health care costs.[29,34,44] Although some studies have found improved outcomes using targeted interventions for depressed high utilizers,[27] there are only a few small studies exploring how costs and utilization after treatment influence outcomes.[45]

Indirect Costs

Not only does depression have a negative impact on overall quality of life, productivity, and earlier life roles (eg, educational attainment, marital timing and stability, and parental function) but it also has a detrimental impact on late life, such as increased days out of life roles, job loss, and diminished financial success.[46] This article provides a concrete example of the indirect costs of depression, namely the relationship between depression and retirement, where adverse consequences may work in both directions.[47] This type of work has previously been conducted in a similar fashion,[7,10] examining the complex bidirectional relations between depression and disability[48] as well as depression and self-rated health.[49]

EXAMPLE: BIDIRECTIONAL RELATIONSHIP BETWEEN DEPRESSION AND RETIREMENT
Background and Introduction

Social and demographic trends, including an aging population, retirement at a younger age, increasing longevity beyond retirement, and an unstable economic climate (potentially leading to involuntary job loss and unplanned earlier or later retirement), highlight the importance of understanding retirement transitions.[50–53] Depression negatively affects labor market activity, including at the retirement transition,[54–59] is associated with substantial functional impairment,[60] and may also be a consequence of retirement transitions.[61–64] Given the centrality of retirement transitions in the lives of older adults, coupled with the implications that these changes have on individuals, their families, employers, the health system, and the US government, there is a need for a comprehensive understanding of the dynamic relationship between depression and retirement and how this relationship may differ across population subgroups. Although some studies suggest that depression may lead to workforce exits, including retirement,[54–56,65] and others indicate that retirement may lead to depression,[66–68] no existing research tests whether and to what extent there are reciprocal influences of depression and retirement and for which groups of people.

Depression can lead to significant functional impairment, and individuals may retire early as a result. Conversely, retirement may lead to feelings of role loss and hence depression. Findings from existing research on the relationship between depression and retirement have produced mixed results. Some studies suggest that workers who become depressed are more likely to retire and retire earlier than desired or planned.[54–56,65] Other studies suggest that once people retire, there is an increased risk of depression,[66–68] although other research indicates that retirement may improve emotional well-being[69–71] and that working in old age may be associated with increased depression.[72,73] Disentangling these relationships can be complex—if people retire early and become depressed, is the depression a cause or a consequence of the retirement timing and decision, or both, or neither? Furthermore, there are a variety of other factors that may influence depression pre-retirement and post-retirement, including age, gender, marital status, race, net worth, physical health, availability of a social support network, other activities such as volunteering, and the sense of meaning and identity that an individual attaches to both working and retiring.

Using an autoregressive cross-lagged panel design and a unique, nationally representative, longitudinal data set of older adults, the authors examined the potentially bidirectional relationship between depression and retirement over time. This research used data from the Health and Retirement Study (HRS), an ongoing study that has examined health, wealth, and retirement biennially among adults aged 50 and older since 1992.[74]

Disciplinary and Theoretic Perspectives

Economists assume that individuals make decisions based on constrained utility maximization. That is, people seek to maximize their lifetime well-being as much as possible given their personal preferences and budgetary or other limitations.[68,75] Individuals trade off consumption during their working lives for consumption in retirement. Consumption in retirement is increased by saving income earned while working, and the amount of the increase depends on the effective savings rate. In theory, people seek to "consumption smooth" across the lifespan, such that consumption across the lifespan is relatively consistent even as earned income is typically volatile, increasing through careers before abruptly dropping at retirement. When individuals act rationally (in economists' sense of the word), their optimal retirement age is determined by this forward-thinking process to ensure maximum well-being throughout their lifespan. There is increasing evidence, however, that people are generally not fully rational in making decisions about savings and retirement.[76] A depressed person may be less able to make optimal decisions about retirement, which may be even more the case if the illness itself impedes rational decision making.[77,78] Furthermore, mental illness may prevent the realization of the optimal timing of retirement, especially if someone needs to leave the workforce early or is unable to return due to depression-related workplace disability. Finally, in a dynamic model over the life course, mental health affects schooling, labor supply, and earnings throughout careers,[79–82] indirectly affecting the ability to optimally time retirement and enjoy retired life.

Disablement theory and stress theory may help explain how depression could lead to retirement. The disablement process describes how chronic and acute conditions (such as depression) affect an individual's functioning as well as factors that accelerate and slow the retirement process,[83,84] potentially necessitating early retirement. In addition, depression may lead to stress, which could negatively affect the immune system response,[85,86] potentially leading to workforce exits. Therefore, it is important to examine the extent to which disablement and stress associated with depression may influence retirement.

Several sociologically based theories, including role theory,[87] life course theory,[62,88,89] and continuity theory[90] could explain how retirement could lead to depression. Retirement viewed as a role exit and a retired person feeling an absence of a new role or identity could lead to depression. Conversely, retirement could improve quality of life for a person seeking or who is satisfied with this new role. For those who prefer continuity to change, retirement could be seen as a disruption and, therefore, lead to emotional distress. However, retirement planned, or viewed as the fulfillment of a goal could be viewed as positive. Finally, if life transitions are viewed in the context of trajectories, and patterns of employment and retirement are viewed as part of the overall life course, then retirement may be positive. Retirement that is disruptive or viewed as "not at the right time," however, could lead to depression.

Although there is less research and theory supporting a simultaneous influence of depression and retirement on each other, it is important to explore all possibilities, including the notion of feedback loops and reciprocal pathways. This type of immediate feedback loop may be more apparent when examining depression and physical comorbidities,[49] but it is likely that with respect to workforce status changes, a time lag of some duration is needed to see how mental health and retirement choices affect each other. Furthermore, comprehensively exploring all possible options for relationships between depression and retirement represents an advance over existing studies.

Methods

Study sample
The authors used HRS data for this study.[74] The HRS is a longitudinal study of a nationally representative cohort of older Americans that was designed to assess the predictors and consequences of transitions out of the workforce in later life. HRS respondents in the analyses met the following criteria: (1) they were born between 1900 and 1947, (2) they were either working or retired in each biennial study wave between 1998 and 2006 (5 total study waves), and (3) they did not have any missing data on any study covariates.

Study measures

Depression Depressive symptom status was measured using the 8-item version of the Center for Epidemiologic Studies Depression Scale (CES-D) to measure depressive symptoms.[91] The CES-D has been used widely in studies of LLD and has good psychometric properties for use in these populations. To determine depressive symptoms, each self-respondent was asked the following questions, with response options of "yes" or "no": (1) Much of the time during the past week, I felt depressed; (2) I felt everything I did was an effort; (3) My sleep was restless; (4) I was happy; (5) I felt lonely; (6) I enjoyed life; (7) I felt sad; and (8) I could not get going. For each respondent, the total number of "yes" responses to questions 1, 2, 3, 5, 7, and 8 and the "no" responses to questions 4 and 6 were summed to arrive at a total depressive symptom score ranging from 0 to 8. Those who reported 4 or more depressive symptoms were classified as having significant depressive symptoms, a cutoff that has been found to produce comparable results to the 16-symptom cutoff for the well-validated 20-item CES-D scale.[92] Given that the CES-D has a well-established second-order factor structure,[49,93] 3 separate additive-composite indicators were created for the present study by summing the responses to the items comprising each dimension (ie, items 1, 6, and 7 for depressive affect; items 2, 3, and 8 for somatic complaints; and items 4 and 6 for positive affect).

Retirement A single binary indicator of employment status was used for this study, based on an indicator of labor force status.[94] If a respondent claimed to be working full time or part time, the respondent was considered "working." If a respondent claimed to be partially retired or fully retired, the respondent was considered "retired." Respondents who claimed to be disabled, unemployed, or not in the labor force were not included.

Covariates The authors included gender, marital status (married/partnered, divorced/separated, widowed, or never married), race/ethnicity (white, black, Hispanic, or other), and level of education (less than high school, high school graduate, or more than high school) as categorical independent variables. Mean age, a count of chronic health conditions (range 0–7), self-assessed health (range 1–5: poor, fair, good, very good, or excellent), functional impairment (range 0–5: none to high), and total household net worth as continuous independent variables in the analyses were included. The 7 possible chronic conditions included (1) high blood pressure or hypertension; (2) diabetes or high blood sugar; (3) cancer or a malignant tumor of any kind except skin cancer; (4) chronic lung disease except asthma, such as chronic bronchitis or emphysema; (5) heart attack, coronary heart disease, angina, congestive heart failure, or other heart problems; (6) stroke or transient ischemic attack; and (7) arthritis or rheumatism (these characteristics are presented in **Table 1**).

Statistical analyses

The authors evaluated the reciprocal relationship between depression and retirement by using an autoregressive cross-lagged panel design with 5 waves of data. Three sets of possible relationships were concurrently tested:

1. Depression leads to retirement.
2. Retirement leads to depression.
3. Depression and retirement occur simultaneously.

Depression and retirement were represented as 10 latent variables: depressive symptomatology (waves 1–5) and retirement (waves 1–5). Each latent variable at

Table 1 Demographic characteristics at 1998 of the HRS cohort sample (n = 8163)[a]	
Characteristic	**Sample (%)**
Gender: female	51.4
Marital status	
Married/partnered	72.4
Divorced/separated	10.9
Widowed	13.8
Never married	3.0
Race/Ethnicity	
White	82.0
Black	11.8
Hispanic	4.6
Other	1.6
Education	
Less than high school	18.9
High school graduate	34.9
More than high school	46.3
Characteristic	**Sample Mean (SD)**
Age (y)	63.8 (8.3)
Number of chronic health conditions (0–7)	1.3 (1.1)
Self-assessed health (1 = poor to 5 = excellent)	2.6 (1.0)
Functional impairment (0 = none to 5 = high)	0.1 (0.5)
Total net worth of assets	$362,193 (754,523)

[a] Sample includes those alive throughout 1998–2006, whose work status was either working or retired at all waves 1998–2006, who did not have any waves of data that were collected by proxy report, and who were born between 1900 and 1947. This included 8175 individuals, of whom 12 were missing data on other covariates.

time (t + 1) is a function of 7 components: first, an autoregression representing the effect of the same variable at the previous time (ie, a 'stability coefficient'); second, the cross-lagged effect of the other latent variable at the previous time; third, a set of time invariant covariates whose regression parameters are allowed to vary across time; fourth, a disturbance for each latent variable that is allowed to correlate with the disturbance for the other latent variable contemporaneously (ie, within the same wave); fifth, 3 indicators for the depression latent variable (depressive affect, somatic complaints, and positive affect), with a given indicator's unstandardized factor loading constrained to be equal across waves; sixth, a single indicator for retirement, with the standardized factor loading set at 1.0 (and thus constrained to be equal across waves); and seventh, an error term for each manifest indicator of the depression latent construct that is allowed to covary with itself across the immediately prior and subsequent wave (ie, autocorrelated measurement errors). The equality constraints on the measurement model (ie, equal factor loadings across waves) comprise an essential assumption that, if not met, precludes testing other parameters in the model.[95] The authors estimated model parameters by using maximum likelihood estimation and used only wave 1 values of the covariates in an attempt to reduce the complexity of the model.

Results

The authors had several notable findings among the 8163 individuals who were either working or retired during the study period (**Fig. 1**).

1. A significant concurrent relationship was found between depression and employment status only at the first wave. This indicated that time lags were needed to help explain the bidirectional relationship between depression and retirement.
2. Second, people who were working compared with those who were retired were found to be significantly less likely to be depressed at the subsequent wave (found in 3 of 4 instances).
3. Finally, depression was found to lead people to be more likely to be retired than working, but this finding was only significant in 1 of 4 instances.

The findings also included relations with covariates primarily in expected directions. Women; black and Hispanic respondents; and those with more comorbid health conditions, activities of daily living limitations, and worse self-assessed health were more likely to be depressed. Those who were more educated, older, married, and of higher net worth were less likely to be depressed. Those with the highest education levels and who were widowed were more likely to be working than retired. Those who were black, who were older, had more health conditions and activities of daily living limitations, had worse self-assessed health, and had higher net worth were less likely to be working than retired. Women, those of other race or Hispanic, and those who were separated or never married were no more likely to be working than retired.

The analyses had several advantages over prior work, because previous studies typically used cross-sectional analyses, had small samples, only focused on 1 of these relationships, used nonrepresentative samples, and used weak measures of mental health or employment status.

Implications of Example for Research and Practice

A key finding from this research is that there is a higher likelihood of depression associated with being retired relative to continuing to work. Furthermore, there was also some evidence that depression may be associated with movement from working status to retirement in the subsequent wave. This research is significant because of the important sociodemographic shifts currently occurring in US society, including an aging population and reductions in labor force growth, an increasing retirement age, pending insolvency of the Social Security system, and medical advances leading to longer life expectancy and declines in physical impairments.[51] In this context, the impact of mental health on quality of life and economic outcomes both pre-retirement and post-retirement may be growing. This research explicitly examined in a longitudinal context how depression and retirement are related. Examining these relationships in a longitudinal, nationally representative sample is a necessary step in determining how best to assist those most at risk for potential negative health and employment outcomes.

PUBLIC HEALTH BURDEN OF LLD

LLD represents a substantial public health burden for older adults,[96] an increasing concern due to the quickly expanding population of elderly in the United States.[10] Although a comprehensive review is beyond the scope of this article, the negative impact that depression has on a wide range of medical conditions and physical impairments is well established.[46,47,97] The presence of depressive disorders often adversely affects the onset,[98] course, and treatment of other chronic diseases.[99,100]

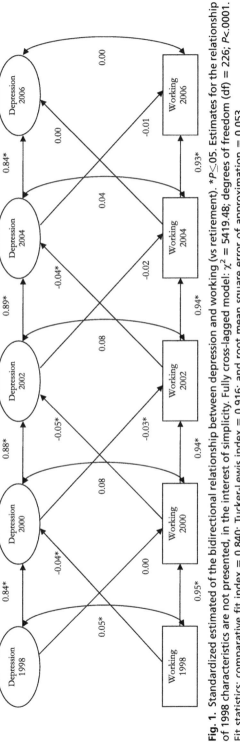

Fig. 1. Standardized estimated of the bidirectional relationship between depression and working (vs retirement). *$P \leq .05$. Estimates for the relationship of 1998 characteristics are not presented, in the interest of simplicity. Fully cross-lagged model: χ^2 = 5419.48; degrees of freedom (df) = 226; $P < .0001$. Fit statistics: comparative fit index = 0.916; Tucker-Lewis index = 0.840; and root mean square error of approximation = 0.053.

Depressed older adults may have multiple complaints.[101] Furthermore, depression may also be associated with unhealthy behaviors and lifestyle choices that exacerbate medical disorders and physical impairments. Therefore, the importance of assessing patients with chronic medical illnesses cannot be overemphasized.[102]

In addition to its impact on physical health, LLD increases the risk of disability,[103] defined as restricting the ability to perform normal activities due to impairment, and of mortality. Depression stands apart as the mental disorder claiming the highest percentage of disability-adjusted life years. Furthermore, analogous to the presence of various patterns of depressive symptoms (discussed previously), depressive symptoms may lead to a variety of patterns of disability over time.[104] Depression is also the mental disorder with the highest increased risk of all-cause mortality[105] and is associated with both all-cause and cause-specific mortality.[106] Finally, LLD has also been shown to decrease active life expectancy.[107]

The depression-mortality hypothesis predicts that depressed people are likely to die sooner than the nondepressed.[108] It suggests that depression and other health conditions indirectly influence each other, leading to a cascade to death.[108] Critics argue that excess natural death (eg, higher rate of mortality beyond expected) in those who are depressed is due to complicating physical illness or poor health behaviors associated with depression rather than depression itself, and that excess deaths are from unnatural causes (ie, suicide).[109] Research suggests that neither suicide nor physical illness nor poor health alone can explain excess mortality among depressed people. Depressive syndromes are associated with significant functional impairment, disability, and suicide. Although most research on depression and mortality has been done in clinical populations,[110] a review of community studies of depression and mortality in older adults found that diagnosed depression was associated with increased mortality.[111] Another recent study also found increased risk of death among older primary care patients with depression.[112]

CAREGIVER BURDEN OF LLD

The negative consequences of LLD, including reduced energy, functioning, and motivation, lead to problems living independently and result in an increased need for unpaid caregiving from friends and family members or informal caregiving.[113] Informal caregiving contributes to the burden of LLD in a several ways. As of 2006, it was estimated that 34 million people provided informal caregiving, the largest source of long-term care in the United States, valued at more than $350 billion annually.[113-115] Caregivers may risk the loss of income, health insurance, and other benefits by giving up or reducing their work hours in order to provide care for depressed loved ones.[113] One study found that depressed elders receive up to 3 additional hours of informal care weekly compared with those without depression, representing a yearly cost of $1330 per person, for a total of more than $9 billion nationwide.[116] This burden encompasses both the value of the care provided and the adverse psychological and physical effects that caregiving has on the informal caregivers themselves.[115,117,118]

Evidence suggests that there are long-term negative health effects and increased mortality risks for those caring for depressed older adults and that caregivers themselves are also likely to suffer from depression.[119] The emotional and physical toll that informal caregiving has on caregivers also affects caregiver family and social network functioning and leads to poorer outcomes and disease trajectories as well as increased use of health care services.[113,120-122] Literature documents the impact affective disorders have on those in a depressed individual's life, especially spouses and partners, family caregivers, and young children who may reside in the household.[114,120,123,124] Recent research suggests that caring for someone with depression is no less burdensome than caring for someone with a schizoaffective disorder or dementia.[122] Additionally, it is possible that there is a mutually reinforcing interaction between caregiver burden and depression and poor outcomes in a care recipient.

Many caregivers report distress. Up to 80% of caregivers endorse issues or treatment of complaints, such as sleep disturbances, depressive symptoms, tension, or fatigue.[120] A high caregiving burden can result in reductions in social or familial support,[120,121] leading to increased vulnerability. Treatment of LLD, however, may mitigate these effects on caregivers and lower overall disease burden.[118]

For young children who reside in the same household as older adults with depression, the impact may be profound. Over time, exposure to a nearby adult with LLD can lead to behavior difficulties, sleep disturbances, school-based problems, attention-deficits, and stunting of social development.[120] Problems that occur in the early stages of life have consequences that can extend beyond the families and individuals touched directly. These issues also affect the health care and welfare systems of the nation over the long term, because childhood-based disturbances may be linked to outcomes ranging from health and well-being to delinquent behavior and lower socioeconomic success.

If the functioning and quality of life of vulnerable older adults suffering from LLD are to improve, the context of these individuals must be considered. Poor prognosis for individuals is intimately tied to their social support networks, and when that support is burdened or impaired, it results in poorer outcomes across the network. The economic burden of LLD is substantial even before considering its long-term impact on the families, children, and caregivers. To improve LLD outcomes, interventions that look beyond depressed individuals must be supported and include partners, friends, children, and other members of an individual's social network.[118]

FUTURE DIRECTIONS
Treatment

Because effective treatments for LLD are available,[125] receiving proper depression care could be beneficial not only for individuals but also for society.[37] Treatment may improve depression outcomes in older adults[126,127] as well as physical functioning.[128,129] Treatments of LLD decrease depression-related costs as well as benefit patients. For example, an intervention of targeted mental health treatment and care coordination reduced costs by accelerating transitions from inpatient to outpatient care, resulting in increased outpatient costs, but nearly tripled the savings in inpatient costs.[130] Although there is substantial evidence documenting the relationship between depression and mortality, there are limited data on how depression treatment might mitigate this effect. Several studies have found that depression treatment and care management decrease mortality[131,132] whereas another study indicated that treatment improves prognosis in community dwelling elderly.[133] Given this promising evidence that treatment may improve outcomes, it may justify increased efforts to prevent, detect, and treat depression.[110] Furthermore, properly addressing the substantial emotional, health, and potential financial needs of depressed older adults could improve quality of life and well-being for these individuals.

Although rates of LLD diagnoses and treatment, particularly with antidepressant medications,[11] have increased over time, many barriers to optimal treatment remain. Depression diagnoses and antidepressant treatment have increased for a variety of reasons, including changes in cultural attitudes, reimbursement practices, and health care delivery.[11] Attributing depression to old age may be a barrier to treatment seeking,[134] and there are many potential reasons for poor treatment adherence in older adults, including stigma, negative patient beliefs about treatment, physical and psychiatric comorbidity, and costs of care.[135] Given that many older patients may prefer psychotherapy over antidepressants,[136] focusing primarily on antidepressants alone represents suboptimal care for LLD. Expanding the availability of promising psychosocial interventions for LLD could be beneficial for patients, caregivers, and society.[11]

Genetics

Another promising area for future research is on genetic contributions to LLD. Genetic explanations, such as gene-environment interactions, may help explain why some individuals become depressed after life changes and others do not.[137] There is debate in the literature regarding the importance of genetic factors on LLD. One explanation suggests that genes may have a less important role in LLD than they do in earlier or childhood-onset depression, positing a more important biologic role, such as vascular explanations, for LLD.[10] An alternative argument suggests that many of the psychosocial factors contributing to earlier life depression, such as family of origin conflicts, have a less important role in later life, leaving a more important role for genetics in the management of mood over the lifespan. Given the limited focus on genetics of LLD (compared with earlier-onset depression),[138] there is substantial room for additional study of both the genetic contributors to LLD and the gene-environment interactions that may lead to either vulnerability or resilience to LLD, which may be related to issues such as loss of independence, spouse or family members, and increased medical illness. It is important to remember, however, that although genetic explanations may be attractive, research indicates that environmental factors explain at least as much of the variance in depression as genes do.[139]

SUMMARY

This article highlights the multiple burdens of LLD on patients, caregivers, and society. Basic, clinical, epidemiologic, and health services research should focus more resources and attention on this devastating and costly yet treatable illness.

ACKNOWLEDGMENTS

The authors would like to acknowledge Amy S.B. Bohnert, PhD; Sharon Maccini, PhD; and Erin M. Miller, MS, for their contributions to earlier versions of this article.

REFERENCES

1. Department of Health and Human Services, Administration on Aging. Older adults and mental health issues and opportunities. Department of Health and Human Services, Washington, DC: Administration on Aging; 2001.
2. Mulsant BH, Ganguli M. Epidemiology and diagnosis of depression in late life. J Clin Psychiatry 1999;60:9–15.
3. Hybels CF, Pieper CF. Epidemiology and geriatric psychiatry. Am J Geriatr Psychiatry 2009;17(8):627–31.
4. Compton WM, Conway KP, Stinson FS, et al. Changes in the prevalence of major depression and comorbid substance use disorders in the United States between 1991-1992 and 2001-2002. Am J Psychiatry 2006;163(12):2141–7.

5. Chapman DP, Perry GS. Depression as a major component of public health for older adults. Prev Chronic Dis 2008;5(1):A22.
6. Gallo JJ, Lebowitz BD. The epidemiology of common late-life mental disorders in the community: themes for the new century. Psychiatr Serv 1999;50(9):1158–66.
7. Institute of Medicine. The mental health and substance use workforce for older adults: in whose hands? Washington, DC: The National Academies Press; 2012.
8. Crystal S, Sambamoorthi U, Walkup JT, et al. Diagnosis and treatment of depression in the elderly medicare population: predictors, disparities, and trends. J Am Geriatr Soc 2003;51(12):1718–28.
9. Valenstein M, Vijan S, Zeber JE, et al. The cost-utility of screening for depression in primary care. Annals of Internal Medicine 2001;134(5):345–60.
10. Beyer JL. Managing depression in geriatric populations. Ann Clin Psychiatry 2007;19(4):221–38.
11. Akincigil A, Olfson M, Walkup JT, et al. Diagnosis and treatment of depression in older community-dwelling adults: 1992-2005. J Am Geriatr Soc 2011;59(6):1042–51.
12. Mitchell AJ, Rao S, Vaze A. Do primary care physicians have particular difficulty identifying late-life depression? A meta-analysis stratified by age. Psychother Psychosom 2010;79(5):285–94.
13. Wu Z, Schimmele CM, Chappell NL. Aging and late-life depression. J Aging Health 2012;24(1):3–28.
14. Luppa M, Luck T, Konig HH, et al. Natural course of depressive symptoms in late life. An 8-year population-based prospective study. J Affect Disord 2012;142(1–3):166–71.
15. Liang J, Xu X, Quinones AR, et al. Multiple trajectories of depressive symptoms in middle and late life: racial/ethnic variations. Psychol Aging 2011;26(4):761–77.
16. Yang Y. Is old age depressing? Growth trajectories and cohort variations in late-life depression. J Health Soc Behav 2007;48(1):16–32.
17. Kuchibhatla MN, Fillenbaum GG, Hybels CF, et al. Trajectory classes of depressive symptoms in a community sample of older adults. Acta Psychiatr Scand 2012;125(6):492–501.
18. Byers A, Vittinghoff E, Lui LY, et al. Twenty-year depressive trajectories among older women. Arch Gen Psychiatry 2012;69(10):1073–9.
19. Hybels CF, Blazer DG, Pieper CF, et al. Profiles of depressive symptoms in older adults diagnosed with major depression: latent cluster analysis. Am J Geriatr Psychiatry 2009;17(5):387–96.
20. Hybels CF, Pieper CF, Blazer DG, et al. The course of depressive symptoms in older adults with comorbid major depression and dysthymia. Am J Geriatr Psychiatry 2008;16(4):300–9.
21. Andreescu C, Chang C, Mulsant B, et al. Twelve-year depressive symptom trajectories and their predictors in a community sample of older adults. Int Psychogeriatr 2008;20(2):221–36.
22. Bogner HR, Morales KH, Reynolds CF, et al. Prognostic factors, course, and outcome of depression among older primary care patients: The PROSPECT study. Aging Ment Health 2012;12(4):452–61.
23. Hall RC, Wise MG. The clinical and financial burden of mood disorders. Cost and outcome. Psychosomatics 1995;36(2):S11–8.
24. Smit F, Cuijpers P, Oostenbrink J, et al. Costs of nine common mental disorders: implications for curative and preventive psychiatry. J Ment Health Policy Econ 2006;9(4):193–200.

25. American Society of Health-System Pharmacists. ASHP therapeutic position statement on the recognition and treatment of depression in older adults. Am J Health Syst Pharm 1998;55(23):2514–8.

26. Beekman AT, Penninx BW, Deeg DJ, et al. The impact of depression on the well-being, disability and use of services in older adults: a longitudinal perspective. Acta Psychiatr Scand 2002;105(1):20–7.

27. Katzelnick DJ, Simon GE, Pearson SD, et al. Randomized trial of a depression management program in high utilizers of medical care. Arch Fam Med 2000; 9(4):345–51.

28. Johnson J, Weissman MM, Klerman GL. Service utilization and social morbidity associated with depressive symptoms in the community. JAMA 1992;267(11): 1478–83.

29. Unutzer J, Patrick DL, Simon G, et al. Depressive symptoms and the cost of health services in HMO patients aged 65 years and older. A 4-year prospective study. JAMA 1997;277(20):1618–23.

30. Katon W, Von Korff M, Lin E, et al. Distressed high utilizers of medical care. DSM-III-R diagnoses and treatment needs. Gen Hosp Psychiatry 1990;12(6): 355–62.

31. Luber MP, Meyers BS, Williams-Russo PG, et al. Depression and service utilization in elderly primary care patients. Am J Geriatr Psychiatry 2001;9(2):169–76.

32. Simon G, Ormel J, VonKorff M, et al. Health care costs associated with depressive and anxiety disorders in primary care. Am J Psychiatry 1995; 152(3):352–7.

33. Manning WG Jr, Wells KB. The effects of psychological distress and psychological well-being on use of medical services. Med Care 1992;30(6):541–53.

34. Simon GE, VonKorff M, Barlow W. Health care costs of primary care patients with recognized depression. Arch Gen Psychiatry 1995;52(10):850–6.

35. Goldney RD, Fisher LJ, Dal Grande E, et al. Subsyndromal depression: prevalence, use of health services and quality of life in an Australian population. Soc Psychiatry Psychiatr Epidemiol 2004;39(4):293–8.

36. Druss BG, Rosenheck RA. Patterns of health care costs associated with depression and substance abuse in a national sample. Psychiatr Serv 1999;50(2): 214–8.

37. Vasiliadis HM, Dionne PA, Preville M, et al. The excess healthcare costs associated with depression and anxiety in elderly living in the community. Am J Geriatr Psychiatry 2013;21(6):536–48.

38. Klinkman MS. Competing demands in psychosocial care. A model for the identification and treatment of depressive disorders in primary care. Gen Hosp Psychiatry 1997;19(2):98–111.

39. Huang BY, Cornoni-Huntley J, Hays JC, et al. Impact of depressive symptoms on hospitalization risk in community-dwelling elder persons. J Am Geriatr Soc 2000;48(10):1279–84.

40. Himelhoch S, Weller WE, Wu AW, et al. Chronic medical illness, depression, and use of acute medical services among Medicare beneficiaries. Med Care 2004; 42(6):512–21.

41. Levenson JL, Hamer RM, Rossiter LF. Relation of psychopathology in general medical inpatients to use and cost of services. Am J Psychiatry 1990;147(11): 1498–503.

42. Unutzer J, Schoenbaum M, Katon WJ, et al. Healthcare costs associated with depression in medically ill fee-for-service medicare participants. J Am Geriatr Soc 2009;57(3):506–10.

43. Katon WJ, Lin E, Russo J, et al. Increased medical costs of a population-based sample of depressed elderly patients. Arch Gen Psychiatry 2003;60(9): 897–903.
44. Rost K, Zhang M, Fortney J, et al. Expenditures for the treatment of major depression. Am J Psychiatry 1998;155(7):883–8.
45. Katzelnick DJ, Kobak KA, Greist JH, et al. Effect of primary care treatment of depression on service use by patients with high medical expenditures. Psychiatr Serv 1997;48(1):59–64.
46. Kessler RC. The costs of depression. Psychiatr Clin North Am 2012;35(1):1–14.
47. Unutzer J, Park M. Public health burden of late-life mood disorders. In: Lavretsky H, Sajatovic M, Reynolds CF 3rd, editors. Late-life mood disorders. New York: Oxford University Press; 2013. p. 42–60.
48. Chen CM, Mullan J, Su YY, et al. The longitudinal relationship between depressive symptoms and disability for older adults: a population-based study. J Gerontol A Biol Sci Med Sci 2012;67(10):1059–67.
49. Kosloski K, Stull DE, Kercher K, et al. Longitudinal analysis of the reciprocal effects of self-assessed global health and depressive symptoms. J Gerontol B Psychol Sci Soc Sci 2005;60(6):P296–303.
50. Gendell M. Retirement age declines again in 1990s. Mon Labor Rev 2001; 124(10):12–21.
51. Mermin GB, Johnson RW, Murphy DP. Why do boomers plan to work longer? J Gerontol B Psychol Sci Soc Sci 2007;62(5):S286–94.
52. Feldman DC. The decision to retire early: a review and conceptualization. Acad Manage Rev 1994;19(2):285–311.
53. Hayward MD, Grady WR, McLaughlin SD. Changes in the retirement process among older men in the United States: 1972-1980. Demography 1988;25(3): 371–86.
54. Conti RM, Berndt ER, Frank RG. Early retirement and public disability insurance applications exploring the impact of depression. Cambridge (MA): National Bureau of Economic Research; 2006.
55. Doshi JA, Cen L, Polsky D. Depression and retirement in late middle-aged U.S. workers. Health Serv Res 2008;43(2):693–713.
56. Karpansalo M, Kauhanen J, Lakka TA, et al. Depression and early retirement: prospective population based study in middle aged men. J Epidemiol Community Health 2005;59(1):70–4.
57. Wray LA. Mental health and labor force exits in older workers the mediating or moderating roles of physical health and job factors. Ann Arbor (MI): University of Michigan; 2003.
58. Waghorn G, Chant D. Receiving treatment and labor force activity in a community survey of people with anxiety and affective disorders. J Occup Rehabil 2007;17(4):623–40.
59. Marcotte DE, Wilcox-Gok V, Redmon PD. Prevalence and patterns of major depressive disorder in the United States labor force. J Ment Health Policy Econ 1999;2(3):123–31.
60. Penninx BW, Deeg DJ, van Eijk JT, et al. Changes in depression and physical decline in older adults: a longitudinal perspective. J Affect Disord 2000; 61(1–2):1–12.
61. Christ SL, Lee DJ, Fleming LE, et al. Employment and occupation effects on depressive symptoms in older Americans: does working past age 65 protect against depression? J Gerontol B Psychol Sci Soc Sci 2007;62(6): S399–403.

62. Kim JE, Moen P. Retirement transitions, gender, and psychological well-being: a life-course, ecological model. J Gerontol B Psychol Sci Soc Sci 2002;57(3): P212–22.

63. Szinovacz ME, Davey A. Retirement transitions and spouse disability: effects on depressive symptoms. J Gerontol B Psychol Sci Soc Sci 2004;59(6): S333–42.

64. Lindeboom M, Portrait F, van den Berg GJ. An econometric analysis of the mental-health effects of major events in the life of older individuals. Health Econ 2002;11(6):505–20.

65. Sobocki P, Lekander I, Borgstrom F, et al. The economic burden of depression in Sweden from 1997 to 2005. Eur Psychiatry 2007;22(3):146–52.

66. Butterworth P, Gill SC, Rodgers B, et al. Retirement and mental health: analysis of the Australian national survey of mental health and well-being. Soc Sci Med 2006;62(5):1179–91.

67. Buxton JW, Singleton N, Melzer D. The mental health of early retirees– national interview survey in Britain. Soc Psychiatry Psychiatr Epidemiol 2005;40(2): 99–105.

68. Charles KK. Is retirement depressing - labor force inactivity and psychological well-being in later life. Cambridge (MA): National Bureau of Economic Research; 2002. p. 9033.

69. Drentea P. Retirement and mental health. J Aging Health 2002;14(2):167–94.

70. Midanik LT, Soghikian K, Ransom LJ, et al. The effect of retirement on mental health and health behaviors: the Kaiser Permanente Retirement Study. J Gerontol B Psychol Sci Soc Sci 1995;50(1):S59–61.

71. Reitzes DC, Mutran EJ, Fernandez ME. Does retirement hurt well-being? Factors influencing self-esteem and depression among retirees and workers. Gerontologist 1996;36(5):649–56.

72. Choi NG, Bohman TM. Predicting the changes in depressive symptomatology in later life: how much do changes in health status, marital and caregiving status, work and volunteering, and health-related behaviors contribute? J Aging Health 2007;19(1):152–77.

73. Mein G. Is retirement good or bad for mental and physical health functioning? Whitehall II longitudinal study of civil servants. J Epidemiol Community Health 2003;57(1):46–9.

74. Juster FT, Suzman R. An overview of the health and retirement study. J Hum Resour 1995;30(Supplement):S7–56.

75. Raymo JM, Sweeney MM. Work-family conflict and retirement preferences. J Gerontol B Psychol Sci Soc Sci 2006;61(3):S161–9.

76. Choi J, Laibson D, Madrian B, et al. Saving for retirement on the path of least resistance. In: McCaffrey E, Slemrod J, editors. Behavioral Public Finance: Toward a New Agenda. New York: Russell Sage Foundation; 2006. p. 304–51.

77. Frank R, McGuire T. Economics and mental health. In: Culyer A, Newhouse J, editors. Handbook of health economics, vol. 1. Philadelphia, PA: Elsevier; 2000. p. 893–954.

78. Frank RG. Behavioral economics and health economics. Cambridge (MA): National Bureau of Economic Research; 2004.

79. Ettner SL, Frank RG, Kessler RC. The impact of psychiatric disorders on labor market outcomes. Ind Labor Relat Rev 1997;51(1):64–81.

80. Timbie JW, Horvitz-Lennon M, Frank RG, et al. A meta-analysis of labor supply effects of interventions for major depressive disorder. Psychiatr Serv 2006;57(2): 212–8.

81. Kessler RC, Frank RG. The impact of psychiatric disorders on work loss days. Psychol Med 1997;27(4):861–73.

82. Kessler RC, Barber C, Birnbaum HG, et al. Depression in the workplace: effects on short-term disability. Health Aff 1999;18(5):163–71.

83. Verbrugge LM, Jette AM. The disablement process. Soc Sci Med 1994;38(1):1–14.

84. Van Gool CH, Kempen GI, Penninx BW, et al. Impact of depression on disablement in late middle aged and older persons: results from the Longitudinal Aging Study Amsterdam. Soc Sci Med 2005;60(1):25–36.

85. Kiecolt-Glaser JK, Glaser R. Depression and immune function: central pathways to morbidity and mortality. J Psychosom Res 2002;53(4):873–6.

86. Kiecolt-Glaser JK, McGuire L, Robles TF, et al. Emotions, morbidity, and mortality: new perspectives from psychoneuroimmunology. Annu Rev Psychol 2002; 53:83–107.

87. George LK. Sociological perspectives on life transitions. Annu Rev Sociol 1993; 19:353–73.

88. Han SK, Moen P. Work and family over time: a life course approach. Ann Am Acad Pol Soc Sci 1999;562:98–110.

89. Szinovacz ME, Davey A. Honeymoons and joint lunches: effects of retirement and spouse's employment on depressive symptoms. J Gerontol B Psychol Sci Soc Sci 2004;59(5):P233–45.

90. Quick HE, Moen P. Gender, employment, and retirement quality: a life course approach to the differential experiences of men and women. J Occup Health Psychol 1998;3(1):44–64.

91. Radloff L. The CES-D scale: a self-report depression scale for research in the general population. Appl Psychol Meas 1977;1(3):385–401.

92. Steffick DE. Documentation of affective functioning measures in the health and retirement study. Ann Arbor (MI): University of Michigan; 2000.

93. Hertzog C, Van Alstine J, Usala PD, et al. Measurement properties of the Center for Epidemiological Studies Depression Scale (CES-D) in older populations. Psychol Assess 1990;2(1):64–72.

94. St Clair P, Blake D, Bugliari D, et al. RAND HRS Data Documentation, Version H. Santa Monica, CA: Labor & Population Program, RAND Center for the Study of Aging; February 2008.

95. Ferrer E, McArdle JJ. Alternative structural models for multivariate longitudinal data analysis. Struct Equ Modeling 2003;10(4):493–524.

96. Lebowitz BD, Pearson JL, Schneider LS, et al. Diagnosis and treatment of depression in late life. Consensus statement update. JAMA 1997;278(14):1186–90.

97. Katon WJ. Clinical and health services relationships between major depression, depressive symptoms, and general medical illness. Biol Psychiatry 2003;54(3):216–26.

98. Karakus MC, Patton LC. Depression and the onset of chronic illness in older adults: a 12-year prospective study. J Behav Health Serv Res 2011;38(3):373–82.

99. Chapman DP, Perry GS, Strine TW. The vital link between chronic disease and depressive disorders. Prev Chronic Dis 2005;2(1):1–10.

100. Murray CJ, Lopez AD, editors. The global burden of disease. Boston: The Harvard School of Public Health; 1996. Global Burden of Disease and Injury Series.

101. Drayer RA, Mulsant BH, Lenze EJ, et al. Somatic symptoms of depression in elderly patients with medical comorbidities. Int J Geriatr Psychiatry 2005; 20(10):973–82.

102. Cyr NC. Depression and older adults. AORN J 2007;85(2):397–401.

103. Carriere I, Gutierrez LA, Peres K, et al. Late life depression and incident activity limitations: influence of gender and symptom severity. J Affect Disord 2011; 133(1–2):42–50.

104. Hybels CF, Pieper CF, Blazer DG, et al. Trajectories of mobility and IADL function in older patients diagnosed with major depression. Int J Geriatr Psychiatry 2010; 25(1):74–81.

105. Eaton WW, Martins SS, Nestadt G, et al. The burden of mental disorders. Epidemiol Rev 2008;30(1):1–14.

106. Lin EH, Heckbert SR, Rutter CM, et al. Depression and increased mortality in diabetes: unexpected causes of death. Ann Fam Med 2009;7(5):414–21.

107. Reynolds SL, Haley WE, Kozlenko N. The impact of depressive symptoms and chronic diseases on active life expectancy in older Americans. Am J Geriatr Psychiatry 2008;16(5):425–32.

108. Schulz R, Martire LM, Beach SR, et al. Depression and mortality in the elderly. Curr Dir Psychol Sci 2000;9(6):204–8.

109. Black DW, Winokur G, Nasrallah A. Is death from natural causes still excessive in psychiatric patients- A follow up of 1593 patients with major-affective disorder. J Nerv Ment Dis 1987;175(11):674–80.

110. Cole MG. Does depression in older medical inpatients predict mortality? A systematic review. Gen Hosp Psychiatry 2007;29(5):425–30.

111. Saz P, Dewey ME. Depression, depressive symptoms and mortality in persons aged 65 and over living in the community: a systematic review of the literature. Int J Geriatr Psychiatry 2001;16(6):622–30.

112. Bogner HR, Morales KH, Reynolds CF, et al. Course of depression and mortality among older primary care patients. Am J Geriatr Psychiatry 2012;20(10): 895–903.

113. Verma K, Silverman BC. Economic burden of late-life depression: cost of illness, cost of treatment, and cost control policies. In: Ellison JM, Kyomen HH, Verma S, editors. Mood disorders in later life. New York: Informa Healthcare; 2009. p. 111–21.

114. Family Caregiver Alliance. Fact sheet: selected caregiver statistics. San Francisco (CA): Family Caregiver Alliance; 2012.

115. Clark MC, Diamond PM. Depression in family caregivers of elders: a theoretical model of caregiver burden, sociotropy, and autonomy. Res Nurs Health 2010; 33(1):20–34.

116. Langa KM, Valenstein MA, Fendrick AM, et al. Extent and cost of informal caregiving for older Americans with symptoms of depression. Am J Psychiatry 2004; 161(5):857–63.

117. Pinquart M, Sorensen S. Differences between caregivers and noncaregivers in psychological health and physical health: a meta-analysis. Psychol Aging 2003; 18(2):250–67.

118. Martire LM, Schulz R, Reynolds CF, et al. Treatment of late-life depression alleviates caregiver burden. J Am Geriatr Soc 2010;58(1):23–9.

119. Thompson A, Fan MY, Unutzer J, et al. One extra month of depression: the effects of caregiving on depression outcomes in the IMPACT trial. Int J Geriatr Psychiatry 2008;23(5):511–6.

120. Van Wijngaarden B, Schene AH, Koeter MW. Family caregiving in depression: impact on caregivers' daily life, distress, and help seeking. J Affect Disord 2004;81(3):211–22.

121. Wang JK, Zhao XD. Family functioning and social support for older patients with depression in an urban area of Shanghai, China. Arch Gerontol Geriatr 2012; 55(3):574–9.

122. Rane LJ, Fekadu A, Papadopoulos AS, et al. Psychological and physiological effects of caring for patients with treatment-resistant depression. Psychol Med 2012;42(9):1825–33.
123. Alzheimer's Association. Facts and figures Alzheimer's disease facts and figures. Chicago, IL: Alzheimer's Association; 2012.
124. National Family Caregivers Association. Caregiver Survey-2000. Kensington (MD): National Family Caregivers Association (NFCA); 2000.
125. Cuijpers P, van Straten A, Smit F. Psychological treatment of late-life depression: a meta-analysis of randomized controlled trials. Int J Geriatr Psychiatry 2006; 21(12):1139–49.
126. Harpole LH, Williams JW Jr, Olsen MK, et al. Improving depression outcomes in older adults with comorbid medical illness. Gen Hosp Psychiatry 2005;27(1): 4–12.
127. Sirey JA, Bruce ML, Alexopoulos GS. The Treatment Initiation Program: an intervention to improve depression outcomes in older adults. Am J Psychiatry 2005; 162(1):184–6.
128. Callahan CM, Kroenke K, Counsell SR, et al. Treatment of depression improves physical functioning in older adults. J Am Geriatr Soc 2005;53(3):367–73.
129. Ciechanowski P, Wagner E, Schmaling K, et al. Community-integrated home-based depression treatment in older adults: a randomized controlled trial. JAMA 2004;291(13):1569–77.
130. Kominski G, Andersen R, Bastani R, et al. UPBEAT: the impact of a psychogeriatric intervention in VA medical centers. Unified Psychogeriatric Biopsychosocial Evaluation and Treatment. Med Care 2001;39(5):500–12.
131. Avery D, Winokur G. Mortality in depressed patients treated with electroconvulsive therapy and antidepressants. Arch Gen Psychiatry 1976;33(9):1029–37.
132. Gallo JJ, Bogner HR, Morales KH, et al. The effect of a primary care practice-based depression intervention on mortality in older adults - A Randomized trial. Ann Intern Med 2007;146(10):689–98.
133. Denihan A, Kirby M, Bruce I, et al. Three-year prognosis of depression in the community-dwelling elderly. Br J Psychiatry 2000;176:453–7.
134. Sarkisian CA, Lee-Henderson MH, Mangione CM. Do depressed older adults who attribute depression to "old age" believe it is important to seek care? J Gen Intern Med 2003;18(12):1001–5.
135. Zivin K, Kales HC. Adherence to depression treatment in older adults: a narrative review. Drugs Aging 2008;25(7):559–71.
136. Unutzer J, Katon W, Callahan CM, et al. Depression treatment in a sample of 1,801 depressed older adults in primary care. J Am Geriatr Soc 2003;51(4): 505–14.
137. Monroe SM, Reid MW. Life stress and major depression. Curr Dir Psychol Sci 2009;18(2):68–72.
138. Kim JM, Stewart R, Kim SW, et al. Interactions between life stressors and susceptibility genes (5-HTTLPR and BDNF) on depression in Korean elders. Biol Psychiatry 2007;62(5):423–8.
139. Tennant C. Life events, stress and depression: a review of recent findings. Aust N Z J Psychiatry 2002;36(2):173–82.

A Team-based Approach to the Care of Depression in Later Life

Where Are We Now?

Jeanne M. Cartier, PhD, PMHCNS-BC, CNE

KEYWORDS

- Team health care • Late life depression • Geriatric depression
- Elderly mental health • Comorbidities • Collaborative care
- Health care workforce development

KEY POINTS

- Major depressive disorder continues to be a leading cause of disability worldwide.
- The elderly population in the United States is continuing to grow at historic rates, increasingly compromising a greater proportion of the population.
- The supply of geriatric practitioners is inadequate to meet the growing needs of the population.
- Collaborative/team-based care models continue to demonstrate the ability to provide effective and efficient care.
- The widespread adoption of team-based care models will require policy change.

INTRODUCTION

The care and the treatment of older adults with depression is a highly relevant social and medical issue. The rapid growth in the number of older adults, a decline in both primary and specialty health care providers, and the functional and financial impact of depression at a national and global level contribute to recognition that current treatment models are likely to be inadequate to meet projected needs. Over the last few decades, other approaches to health care have been found to be effective in demonstration projects. However, to date there has been little widespread adoption of these approaches. This article reviews briefly the historical genesis of collaborative and team-based models of care, including the results of projects that have been reported through the mid 2000s. A more comprehensive review of research and project

Funding Sources: Nil.
Conflict of Interest: Nil.
Department of Biobehavioral Nursing, College of Nursing, Georgia Regents University, 1120 15th Street, EC 4348, Augusta, GA 30912, USA
E-mail address: jcartier@gru.edu

Psychiatr Clin N Am 36 (2013) 651–660
http://dx.doi.org/10.1016/j.psc.2013.08.009
0193-953X/13/$ – see front matter © 2013 Elsevier Inc. All rights reserved.

outcomes published during the last 5 years on this model of care addressing either depression or depression with comorbid conditions follows. Reported outcomes include not only health outcome indicators per se but also evidence related to patient and provider satisfaction. Last, the move to a new model of care is discussed. With the Patient Protection and Accountable Care Act of 2010 and the establishment of medical homes, it is likely that eventually a team-based or some type of collaborative care is likely to become the norm. Challenges to current and future practices, especially those associated with full implementation of this model, are identified. Finally, implications for practice, education, and research are addressed.

THE AGING POPULATION

The elderly population (65 years or older) in the United States has experienced rapid growth in the last decade and will soon eclipse all previous numbers in both number and percentage of the population. According to the US Census Bureau,[1] in the last decade the rate of increase in the elderly has increased by 15.1% with 40.3 million elders in the Unites States as of April 2010. The number of elderly will continue to increase as baby boomers age, resulting in the older population comprising a great proportion of the total population.

MENTAL HEALTH AND DEPRESSION

Depression continues to be a significant contributor to the burden of disease worldwide. In the most recent study of the global burden of disease,[2] mental and behavioral conditions constitute a major part of the burden across all regions of the world with the exception of high-income Asian Pacific and South Asia; together they account for 22.7% of years lived with disability. Major depressive disorders is the leading cause contributing 8.1% of total years lived with disability by itself; among all causes of disability major depressive disorder ranks second only to low back pain.

Depression diagnoses among older adults in the United States have increased over the last 20 years. Analysis of Medicare data from 1992 to 2005 reports that over the 10-year period rates of depression doubled to 6.3% in community-dwelling fee-for-service Medicare beneficiaries.[3]

HEALTH CARE WORKFORCE

The rapid increase in the aging population will increase the demand for geriatric practitioners. The Institute of Medicine (IOM)[4] has dubbed this great surge of the aging population "the silver tsunami" because it will overwhelm a workforce that will be inadequate to provide general health care or specialty services. The inadequacy exists both for geriatric providers and for geriatric psychiatric providers. Although current elders are often treated within a geriatric practice, it is hypothesized that as baby boomers age, they will continue to seek out mental health care from psychiatric clinicians,[4] amplifying the need to have providers capable of treating mental health disorders, especially depression and anxiety. Although advanced practice registered nurses and geriatric nurse practitioners are educated and trained and could potentially increase the pool of geriatric and geriatric mental health care providers, in many states their practice is restricted by law.[5] A major recommendation from the Robert Wood Johnson Foundation/IOM report on the future of nursing was that legislative barriers and restrictions should be removed in order for advanced practice nurses "to practice to the full extent of their education and training."[5]

Another barrier to providing care to the older adult with depression is bureaucratic policies related to reimbursement. There is ample evidence that suggests that older adults with depression are best treated with outreach, screening, monitoring, and education and support,[4] yet many current practices and payers' will reimburse disease-specific outcomes and procedures and not multidimensional or integrated care.

One of the ways for the health care system to respond to this overwhelming need is to provide care services that not only are efficient and make best use of limited resources but also are effective in that health outcomes are positive and exceed current outcomes associated with usual care practices. Through several demonstration and grant programs, team-based care has provided such a model.

HISTORICAL PERSPECTIVE OF THE CHRONIC CARE MODEL

The chronic care model was developed by Wagner in the 1990s with a goal of providing quality medical care to chronically ill people.[6] The idea of providing care to chronically ill or vulnerable people was not new; there was a precedent for providing programs of care for special populations such as the mentally ill, homeless, and elderly. However, unlike those initiatives that were designed and limited to meet population-specific needs, Wagner was charged with developing a model that would meet needs across chronic care conditions. The chronic care model underwent extensive testing and refinement. In 2001, Wagner and colleagues[7] identified 6 guiding elements of the model to guide quality care and improved health outcomes. The first Congress on Improving Chronic Care[8] was held in 2002 and focused on quality improvement. Many of the major issues and ideas presented at that first congress continue to be part of collaborative care projects and the subject of research interventions. Specifically, those ideas included "stepped intervention, multi-component interventions, reimbursement that rewards quality care, trained providers and activated patients, cultural competence and patient centered care."[8]

RECENT RESEARCH ON COLLABORATIVE CARE MODELS TREATING DEPRESSION ALONE

For this article, an electronic search of the databases and hand searching were conducted to identify continued evidence on the effectiveness of collaborative care models. Because there is a paucity of research on collaborative care models specifically designed for older adults, studies were not excluded based on age of participants in the study. The results included not only reports of single condition projects but also included complex patients treated in both primary and specialty settings. The studies were primarily random clinical trials, although implementation and quality improvement projects were also identified. The effectiveness of collaborative care was not limited to the United States; there is a growing body of evidence from Europe that report favorable outcomes relative to collaborative care. A few studies were found that examined patient and provider satisfaction.

To date, there have been at least 2 systematic reviews evaluating depression outcomes associated with the collaborative care model. The first systematic review[9] identified 37 published studies from 1993 through 2004; the second[10] evaluated an additional 32 studies published through 2009. Studies included in both of these were predominantly random clinical trials. Results from both of these reviews support collaborative care as an effective treatment approach to depression. Compared with usual care, the positive outcomes associated with collaborative care included depression symptom improvement, adherence, response to treatment, and remission. Additional analysis in the second review revealed that registered nurse case managers exerted a greater effect on outcomes compared with case managers from other backgrounds.

There are few studies that are limited exclusively to collaborative care for older adults with depression. In one such study, the investigators examined whether there was a differential response to this model of care relative to age. In this large (N = 906) multisite randomized trial the young-old and old-old were compared on depression symptoms, treatment response, and remission.[11] Results indicate the initial response did not differ based on age. Although both groups trended downward over time, the old-old had significantly lower rates of response and remission rates when compared with the young-old. The investigators suggest further studies are needed to understand the difference better in long-term outcomes.

One of the most innovative programs focused primarily on treating of geriatric patients with depression is the BRIGTHEN (Bridging Resources of an Interdisciplinary Geriatric Health Team via Electronic Networking) Program.[12] This feasibility study evaluated the ability of a virtual interdisciplinary team to help provide depression treatment and a broad range of services to depressed older adults who might otherwise have difficulty accessing these services. Patients are able to receive services at their usual place of health care. Because the collaboration takes place electronically, the interdisciplinary team is able to support and make recommendations to a greater number primary care and specialists in greater number than if a face-to-face meeting was required. The virtual collaboration makes it possible to include a wide variety of professionals to consider all aspects of the patients' condition and health that may be contribute to improving health outcomes. Interestingly, this is one of the few studies in which the team did not include a nurse. The primary care or specialist provider conducts the initial screening and follow-up assessment if needed. For those patients screened in and willing to participate, the primary care provider distributes the full assessment and report; each member of the team responds with recommendations. The primary care provider then works with the patient to tailor a plan of care and provide referrals as needed. At 6 months participants demonstrated significant (P<.001) improvement as measured by the geriatric depression scale and the Medical Outcomes study-short form 12, mental component. Team members evaluated the program finding the communication process to work well. This model has the potential to expand geriatric mental health specialty care to a broad population.

The Translating Initiatives for Depression into Effective Solutions (TIDES) model of collaborative care was designed and tested as a demonstration project within the Veterans' Affairs system to provide collaborative depression care within the primary care setting.[13] The team consists primarily of mental health registered nurses; a part-time clinical nurse specialist and a consulting psychiatrist provide supervision as needed. Intervention is delivered via telephone over a period of 6 months. The goal of the TIDES program is to improve symptoms, prevent relapse, and encourage treatment adherence through case management activities. This TIDES demonstration project was successful—adherence to medication and follow-up visits, an improvement in depression and functional status scores, and recovery were all achievable within the primary care setting. In addition to the improved health outcomes, patients avoided long waits for referrals and were able to access follow-up in a convenient manner.

Results from at least one randomized controlled trial (RCT)[14] suggest that the collaborative care model may provide better treatment response especially for depressed minority clients. At the conclusion of a 6-month intervention, largely consisting of phone contact by nurses and clinical pharmacists, the minority clients who had received the intervention were more than 6 times more likely to have a response to treatment compared with their Caucasian counterparts (P = .004), whereas there was no disparity in the usual care arm of the study. This strength of this finding continued to exist even when adjusting for other variables.

Globally, there is limited research regarding collaborative and team-based care. In a year-long RCT conducted at 20 primary care centers in Spain, a multicomponent intervention included the inclusion of a nurse as case manager along with educational programming and the use of clinical guidelines.[15] Depression-free days was the outcome variable of interest; it was measured at baseline, and at 3, 6, and 12 months. From the start to end of the study, the mean of depression-free days was 44.1 days higher in the intervention group compared with the usual care group ($P = .001$) intervention group.

RECENT RESEARCH ON COLLABORATIVE CARE OF DEPRESSION WITH COMORBID ILLNESSES

There is a growing body of evidence that suggests the integrated care of depression can be successfully managed in specialty as well as primary care practices. Pyne and colleagues[16] conducted a single-blind randomized clinical effectiveness trial at 3 Veterans' Affairs HIV clinics. The care team for the HIV Translating Initiatives for Depression into Effective Solutions intervention included a registered nurse depression care manager, pharmacist, and psychiatrist. This team, located off-site of the HIV clinic, provided support and treatment recommendations to on-site clinicians via electronic medical records. In addition, the depression care manager communicated with patients via telephone. Treatment followed a stepped-care model; the frequency of contact between the depression care manager and patient was based on the "step" of care being provided. The results supported this approach as effective and cost-effective. However, unlike other studies that demonstrate both initial and sustained differences between the usual care and intervention groups, in this study the intervention group demonstrated a stronger response rate only at the 6-month measurement.

Adams and colleagues[17] also focused on treating comorbid depression in an HIV population. They also used depression care managers and demonstrated the usefulness of algorithms to provide effective antidepressant treatment in an HIV clinic. Nonphysician depression care managers are able to use these evidence-based guidelines (in conjunction with weekly supervision by psychiatrists) to manage these clients with complex needs.

Lin and colleagues[18] conducted an RCT for patients with either poorly controlled diabetes or heart disease and an existing comorbid depression. Nurse care managers were used to coordinate and collaborate with primary care physicians. Nurses engaged with patients to help patients establish goals and teach self-management skills. During the early part of the intervention nurses might have contact with the patient 2 to 3 times a month through either visits or phone calls. As patients became more adept at following through with self-care activities, maintenance plans were jointly established with patients. The frequency of contact by nurse to patient was a function of patients' ability to self-manage. At the end of the 1-year study, patients who were involved in the intervention arm of the study significantly outperformed the usual care arm with respect to the self-management activities of monitoring blood pressure ($P<.001$) and glucose ($P = .06$). With respect to initiation or adjustment of medications, the intervention group consistently and significantly outperformed the usual care group. The highest treatment adjustment was for antidepressants for those in the intervention group; their rate was 6 times the rate of usual care ($P<.01$).

The comorbid presentation of diabetes mellitus and depression is well known. Improvements in either condition are likely to exert a positive health effect on the other. A randomized control study was conducted to test whether an integrated approach to treating both of these conditions was more effective than usual care in adherence to pharmacotherapy regimen for each condition, depression symptom amelioration, and lower glycated hemoglobin levels.[19] The intervention was conducted by either a master's or a bachelor's trained research assistant; total intervention time required for each participant over the course of 3 months was 2 hours total. This brief, rather low-intensity intervention, produced statistically significant improvement. Compared with the usual care group, changes from baseline in the intervention were significant in all 4 outcome variables ($P<.001$).

By design, most of the recent research trials and projects limit outcomes analysis to a single year time point. Ell and coworkers[20] conducted a follow-up study on patients in a previous trial that evaluated collaborative care for depression in patients with cancer; outcome measurements were conducted at 18 and 24 months. This trial was also one of the few focused on low-income and predominantly Hispanic patients. At the endpoint of the first trial, patients receiving the intervention had significantly better outcomes with respect to receiving treatment, to depression symptom reduction, and better quality of life. Results indicated that intervention patients continued to have significantly better outcomes related to quality of life and depression symptoms. However, there was no significant difference between the 2 groups with respect to recurrence or receipt of treatment.

STUDIES RELATED TO PATIENT AND PROVIDER SATISFACTION

Satisfaction with care from both a patient and a provider perspective may directly or indirectly impact treatment adherence and outcomes, yet there is a paucity of literature that examines this variable. In one of the few studies on treating depression in the context of a comorbid illness, both patients and providers indicated a preference for treatment by the general practitioner in a primary care clinic.[21] Although patients and providers had similar preferences for treatment providers and location, they differed on treatment options; patients indicated a preference for "talk treatment," whereas the general practitioners preferred a combination of medication and talk treatment. Limitations for this study included a small sample size (N = 100 patients, 86 general practitioners), a cross-sectional survey design, and sampling from a single center. The study was conducted in England, which further limits generalizability to care in the United States. Despite the limitations and inability to generalize the findings, the study raises awareness of considering satisfaction in planning treatment services. The results from a qualitative study (also conducted in England) exploring patients' experiences with collaborative care indicated that patients found collaborative care to be acceptable and useful.[22]

MOVING TOWARD A NEW MODEL
Implications for Practice

Until such time that collaborative models of care are financially supported and reimbursed, it is unlikely that they will become the norm. However, there are guiding elements and successful strategies within those models that can be adapted to current practice settings. First, practice settings can make deliberate efforts to be patient centric and actively engage patients in their own care. Treatment options and preferences of patients should be considered in making recommendations; when preferences match recommendations, it is likely that there will be greater treatment adherence. Research has demonstrated that older adults' preferences are often not considered.[23] Setting goals that are patient defined, motivational interviewing, coaching, and providing education all can be accomplished within the confines of current practice environments. Identifying community resources either through pamphlets and bulletin boards or on practice Web sites (if available) can help link patients to potential places/activities that will help them in self-management strategies.

The expected burgeoning growth of electronic medical records and other forms of health information technology[24] may create an opportunity for nurses and other health care professionals to be more engaged and health promotion and disease prevention activities.

There are a variety of ways that depression care can be provided from screening to treatment. Based on a large systematic review of the benefits and harms of screening for depression,[25] the US Preventative Task Force recommends screening adults for when staff-assisted depression care supports are in place.[26] However, based on availability of resources, practice sites could determine if they have the ability to pilot small programs using telephone monitoring. Last, primary care clinicians can identify a mental health specialist with whom they can consult with concerning challenging or questionable cases.

Implications for Research

The almost 20 years of research on collaborative care in the treatment of depression provides robust evidence to support it as an effective treatment modality. Research in the last 5 years has expanded to begin to examine the effectiveness in specialty clinics and people with comorbid conditions. There is a limited but growing research base examining some of the cultural factors related to the effectiveness. Thota and colleagues[10] identified several characteristics associated with collaborative care models deserving of further exploration and to date have not been fully explored. These characteristics include further evaluation of both the type of case manager and the training to provide optimal results; identifying the optimal dosing frequency and intensity of case management strategies; expanding knowledge about how this model works beyond the inpatient and outpatient settings in a variety of community settings; and conducting additional studies outside the United States. Cost containment as well as efficacy should be dual goals; although most of the research demonstrates the intervention arm as superior to usual care, perhaps the next step should be 3-armed studies (head-to-head interventions plus usual care). Knowing whether brief low-intensity interventions can perform as well as more involved interventions can be important in planning both efficient and cost-effective care. Translational research to understand better the right mix of providers needed in caring for the elderly depressed population is also needed.

Finally, longitudinal studies are needed to evaluate whether health care outcomes can be sustained over time or if "booster" sessions are warranted. Collectively, current research results to date demonstrate a trend of gradual decline in health outcomes approximately 6 months after the end of interventional trials. Investigation into the composition, timing, and frequency of "booster" sessions may allow clinicians to maximize outcomes over time.

Implications for Education

There is a need for education of geriatric mental health providers at all levels of preparation and across all levels of care. With or without collaborative models of care, health care providers can better serve clients if they are prepared with team skills. Interdisciplinary education and team-based learning are mechanisms by which individuals from a variety of professional backgrounds can learn to become knowledgeable of each other's scope of responsibilities and skill set. Interdisciplinary education should include not only didactic experiences but also clinical training. Health care professionals should receive education and training in team building, collaborating and negotiating skills, and team science. Geriatric competencies have recently been established for nursing curricula at both the bachelor's and the master's level. Core geriatric competencies should be established for all geriatric health care workers. Continuing education programs and staff development training programs can be developed to ensure existing providers have requisite skills.

Educational training can also be targeted at increasing the knowledge and skill level of ancillary workers. These individuals can be trained in the use of coaching and supportive techniques that may help support patients in self-management activities. An educated and skilled ancillary workforce can potentially take on some case management and monitoring activities, freeing up primary and specialty health care providers to take on more complex tasks. Compton[27] has suggested that peer specialists may be able to also fulfill some of these activities. The required knowledge, skills, and training recommended for mental health, substance abuse, and geriatric care from direct care worker to psychiatrist are outlined in the IOM report.[4]

SUMMARY

For more than 20 years various organizations have called for an organizational change to the health care delivery system. This call has been supported by a plethora of robust studies that provide evidence strongly supporting both clinical and cost-effectiveness of various collaborative care models. Until such time that there is a financial incentive rather than disincentive for using a collaborative care approach, it is unlikely that it will become a widespread practice. As health care providers, we can begin to incorporate known successful strategies into our practice while actively advocating for health policy changes.

REFERENCES

1. Werner CA. The older population 2010. 2010 census brief. U.S. Census Bureau C 2010BR-09 November 1 2011. Available at: http://www.census.gov/prod/cen2010/briefs/c2010br-09.pdf. Accessed January 25, 2013.
2. Vos T, Flaxman D, Nughavi M, et al. Years lived with disability (YLDs) for 1160 sequelae of 289 diseases and injuries 1990-2110: a systematic analysis for the global burden of disease study 2010. Lancet 2012;380(9859):2163–96 Retrieved electronically from: http://phstwlp1.partners.org:2139/10.1016/S0140-6736(12)62133-3. Accessed January 20, 2013.
3. Ackincigil A, Olfson M, Walku JT, et al. Diagnosis and treatment of depression in older community-dwelling adults: 1992-2005. J Am Geriatr Soc 2011;59(6):1042–51.
4. IOM (Institute of Medicine). The mental health and substance abuse workforce for older adults: in whose hands? Washington, DC: The National Academies Press; 2012.
5. Committee on the Robert Wood Johnson Foundation Initiative on the future of nursing at the IOM. The future of nursing: leading change, advancing health. Washington, DC: The National Academies Press; 2011. Available at: http://www.nap.edu/catalog/12956.html.
6. Wielawski IM. Improving chronic illness care. In: Isaacs SL, Kickman JR, editors. Chapter three, excerpted from the Robert Wood Johnson foundation anthology: to improve health and health care, vol. X. Princeton (NJ): Robert wood Johnson Foundation; 2006. Available at: http://www.improvingchroniccare.org/downloads/rwjf_anthology_icic.pdf. Accessed February 4, 2013.

7. Wagner EH, Austin BT, Davis C, et al. Improving chronic illness care: translating evidence into action. Health Aff (Millwood) 2001;20(6):64–78.

8. Congress on Improving Chronic Care. Summary of Congress. 2002. Available at: http://www.improvingchroniccare.org/downloads/2002_summary_copy2.pdf. Accessed January 19, 2013.

9. Gilbody S, Bower P, Richards D, et al. Collaborative care for depression: a systematic review and cumulative meta-analysis. Arch Intern Med 2006;166: 2314–21.

10. Thota AB, Sipe TA, Byard GJ, et al. Collaborative care to improve the management of depressive disorders: a community guide systematic review and meta-analysis. Am J Prev Med 2012;42(5):525–38.

11. Williams EV, Unützer J, Lee S, et al. Collaborative depression care for the old-old: finding from the IMPACT trial. J Geriatr Psychiatry 2009;17:1040–9.

12. Emery EE, Lapidos S, Eisenstein AR, et al. The BRIGHTEN program: implementation and evaluation of a program to bridge resources of an interdisciplinary geriatric health team via electronic networking. Gerontologist 2012;52(6):857–65.

13. Machado RJ, Tomlinson V. Bridging the gap between primary care and mental health. J Psychosoc Nurs Ment Health Serv 2011;49(11):24–9.

14. Davis TD, Deen T, Bryant-Bedell K, et al. Does minority racial-ethnic status moderate outcomes of collaborative care for depression. Psychiatr Serv 2011;62:1282–8.

15. López-Cortacans G, Rafecas WB, Alias AC, et al. Effectiveness of a programme for the multidisciplinary approach to depression that boost the nurse's role in primary care [abstract]. Metas de enfermería 2012;15(2):28–32.

16. Pyne JM, Fortney JC, Curran GM, et al. Effectiveness of collaborative care for depression in human immunodeficiency virus clinics. Arch Intern Med 2011; 171(1):23–31.

17. Adams JL, Gaynes BN, McGuinness T, et al. Treating depression within the HIV "Medical Home": a guided algorithm for antidepressant management by HIV clinicians. AIDS Patient Care STDS 2012;26(11):647–54.

18. Lin EH, Von Korff M, Ciechanowski P, et al. Treatment adjustment and medication adherence for complex patients with diabetes, heart disease, and depression: a randomized controlled trial. Ann Fam Med 2012;10(1):6–14.

19. Bogner HR, Moreales KH, de Vries HF, et al. Integrated management of Type 2 diabetes mellitus and depression treatment to improve medication adherence: a randomized controlled trial. Ann Fam Med 2012;10:15–22.

20. Ell K, Xie B, Kapetanovic S, et al. One-year follow-up of collaborative depression care for low-income, predominantly Hispanic patients with cancer. Psychiatr Serv 2011;62:162–70. http://dx.doi.org/10.1176/appi.ps.62.2.162. Available at: http://ps.psychiatryonline.org/article.aspx?article ID=102180. Accessed January 28, 2013.

21. Hodges L, Butcher I, Kleiboer A, et al. Patient and general practitioner preferences for the treatment of depression in patients with cancer: how, who, and where? J Psychosom Res 2009;67:399–402.

22. Simpson A, Richards D, Gask L, et al. Patients' experiences of receiving collaborative care for the treatment of depression in the UK: a qualitative investigation. Ment Health Fam Med 2008;5:95–104.

23. Skultety KM, Rodriqguez RL. Treating geriatric depression in primary care. Curr Psychiatry Rep 2008;10:44–50.

24. Sochalski J, Weiner J. Health care system reform and the nursing workforce: matching practice and skills to future needs, not demands. Appendix F. In: Committee on the Robert Wood Johnson Foundation Initiative on the future of nursing

at the IOM. The future of nursing: leading change, advancing health. Washington, DC: The National Academies Press; 2011. p. 375–400. Available at: http://www. nap.edu/catalog/12956.html.

25. O'Connor EA, Whitlock EP, Beil TL, et al. Screening for depression in adult patients in primary care settings: a systematic evidence review. Ann Intern Med 2009;151:793–803.

26. U.S. Preventative Task Force. Screening for depression in adults: U.S. preventative services task force recommendation statement. Ann Intern Med 2009;151: 784–92.

27. Compton MT. Systemic organizational change for the collaborative care approach to managing depressive disorders. Am J Prev Med 2012;42(5):553–5.

Index

Note: Page numbers of article titles are in **boldface** type.

Psychiatr Clin N Am 36 (2013) 661–669
http://dx.doi.org/10.1016/S0193-953X(13)00113-5
0193-953X/13/$ – see front matter © 2013 Elsevier Inc. All rights reserved.

psych.theclinics.com

United States Postal Service
Statement of Ownership, Management, and Circulation
(All Periodicals Publications Except Requestor Publications)

1. Publication Title
Psychiatric Clinics of North America

2. Publication Number
0 0 0 — 7 0 3

3. Filing Date
9/14/13

4. Issue Frequency
Mar, Jun, Sep, Dec

5. Number of Issues Published Annually
4

6. Annual Subscription Price
$286.00

7. Complete Mailing Address of Known Office of Publication *(Not printer) (Street, city, county, state, and ZIP+4®)*
Elsevier Inc.
360 Park Avenue South
New York, NY 10010-1710

Contact Person
Stephen R. Bushing

Telephone *(Include area code)*
215-239-3688

8. Complete Mailing Address of Headquarters or General Business Office of Publisher *(Not printer)*
Elsevier Inc., 360 Park Avenue South, New York, NY 10010-1710

9. Full Names and Complete Mailing Addresses of Publisher, Editor, and Managing Editor *(Do not leave blank)*

Publisher *(Name and complete mailing address)*
Linda Belfus, Elsevier, Inc., 1600 John F. Kennedy Blvd. Suite 1800, Philadelphia, PA 19103-2899

Editor *(Name and complete mailing address)*
Joanne Husovski, Elsevier, Inc., 1600 John F. Kennedy Blvd. Suite 1800, Philadelphia, PA 19103-2899

Managing Editor *(Name and complete mailing address)*
Barbara Cohen - Kligerman, Elsevier, Inc., 1600 John F. Kennedy Blvd. Suite 1800, Philadelphia, PA 19103-2899

10. Owner *(Do not leave blank. If the publication is owned by a corporation, give the name and address of the corporation immediately followed by the names and addresses of all stockholders owning or holding 1 percent or more of the total amount of stock. If not owned by a corporation, give the names and addresses of the individual owners. If owned by a partnership or other unincorporated firm, give its name and address as well as those of each individual owner. If the publication is published by a nonprofit organization, give its name and address.)*

Full Name	Complete Mailing Address
Wholly owned subsidiary of	1600 John F. Kennedy Blvd, Ste. 1800
Reed/Elsevier, US holdings	Philadelphia, PA 19103-2899

11. Known Bondholders, Mortgagees, and Other Security Holders Owning or Holding 1 Percent or More of Total Amount of Bonds, Mortgages, or Other Securities. If none, check box. ☐ None

Full Name	Complete Mailing Address
N/A	

12. Tax Status *(For completion by nonprofit organizations authorized to mail at nonprofit rates) (Check one)*
The purpose, function, and nonprofit status of this organization and the exempt status for federal income tax purposes:
☐ Has Not Changed During Preceding 12 Months
☐ Has Changed During Preceding 12 Months *(Publisher must submit explanation of change with this statement)*

PS Form 3526, September 2007 (Page 1 of 3 (Instructions Page 3)) PSN 7530-01-000-9931 **PRIVACY NOTICE:** See our Privacy policy in www.usps.com

---

13. Publication Title
Psychiatric Clinics of North America

14. Issue Date for Circulation Data Below
September 2013

15.	Extent and Nature of Circulation		Average No. Copies Each Issue During Preceding 12 Months	No. Copies of Single Issue Published Nearest to Filing Date
a.	Total Number of Copies *(Net press run)*		763	700
b. Paid Circulation (By Mail and Outside the Mail)	(1)	Mailed Outside-County Paid Subscriptions Stated on PS Form 3541. *(Include paid distribution above nominal rate, advertiser's proof copies, and exchange copies)*	381	357
	(2)	Mailed In-County Paid Subscriptions Stated on PS Form 3541 *(Include paid distribution above nominal rate, advertiser's proof copies, and exchange copies)*		
	(3)	Paid Distribution Outside the Mails Including Sales Through Dealers and Carriers, Street Vendors, Counter Sales, and Other Paid Distribution Outside USPS®	160	177
	(4)	Paid Distribution by Other Classes Mailed Through the USPS (e.g. First-Class Mail®)		
c.	Total Paid Distribution *(Sum of 15b (1), (2), (3), and (4))*	▲	541	534
d. Free or Nominal Rate Distribution (By Mail and Outside the Mail)	(1)	Free or Nominal Rate Outside-County Copies Included on PS Form 3541	70	66
	(2)	Free or Nominal Rate In-County Copies Included on PS Form 3541		
	(3)	Free or Nominal Rate Copies Mailed at Other Classes Through the USPS (e.g. First-Class Mail)		
	(4)	Free or Nominal Rate Distribution Outside the Mail (Carriers or other means)		
e.	Total Free or Nominal Rate Distribution (Sum of 15d (1), (2), (3) and (4))	▲	70	66
f.	Total Distribution (Sum of 15c and 15e)		611	600
g.	Copies not Distributed *(See instructions to publishers #4 (page 63))*	▲	152	100
h.	Total (Sum of 15f and g)	▲	763	700
i.	Percent Paid (15c divided by 15f times 100)	▲	88.54%	89.00%

16. Publication of Statement of Ownership
☐ If the publication is a general publication, publication of this statement is required. Will be printed in the December 2013 issue of this publication.
☐ Publication not required

17. Signature and Title of Editor, Publisher, Business Manager, or Owner

(signature) Stephen R. Bushing

Stephen R. Bushing – Inventory Distribution Coordinator

Date September 14, 2013

I certify that all information furnished on this form is true and complete. I understand that anyone who furnishes false or misleading information on this form or who omits material or information requested on the form may be subject to criminal sanctions (including fines and imprisonment) and/or civil sanctions (including civil penalties).

PS Form 3526, September 2007 (Page 2 of 3)

.

Moving?

Make sure your subscription moves with you!

To notify us of your new address, find your **Clinics Account Number** (located on your mailing label above your name), and contact customer service at:

Email: journalscustomerservice-usa@elsevier.com

800-654-2452 (subscribers in the U.S. & Canada)
314-447-8871 (subscribers outside of the U.S. & Canada)

Fax number: 314-447-8029

Elsevier Health Sciences Division
Subscription Customer Service
3251 Riverport Lane
Maryland Heights, MO 63043

*To ensure uninterrupted delivery of your subscription,
please notify us at least 4 weeks in advance of move.

Printed and bound by CPI Group (UK) Ltd, Croydon, CR0 4YY

03/10/2024

01040489-0002